Breast Cancer Diet Cookbook For Beginners

101 Essentially well balanced and easy recipes for supporting overall health during breast cancer treatment and recuperation.

By

Andrea T. Rockwell

Copyright/ Disclaimer

indirect, resulting from the use of the material included in this book is disclaimed by the author and publisher.

All efforts have been taken to guarantee that the data in this book is correct as of the date of release. However, regardless of whether mistakes or omissions are the product of carelessness, an accident, or any other reason, the author and publisher do not assume and hereby disclaim any duty to any party for any loss, damage, or disruption caused by errors or omissions.

We appreciate your observance of the copyright and legal rights pertaining to this book.

About the Author

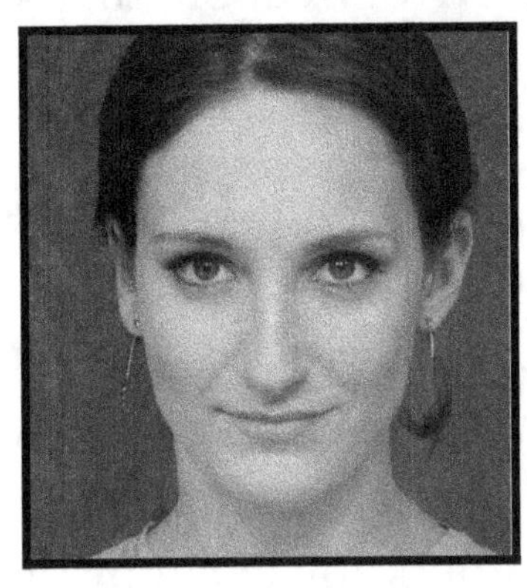

Prolific supporter of health and well-being, Andrea T. Rockwell, puts her knowledge in the spotlight in "Breast Cancer Diet Cookbook For Beginners." Driven by a strong belief in enabling others via education, Andrea has devoted her studies to assisting others in navigating the intricate connection between nutrition and breast cancer.

Throughout the whole book, Andrea's dedication to closing the gap between nutritional study and real-world application is clear. Her work blends a plethora of factual information from studies with a sympathetic awareness of the difficulties experienced by those who have just received a breast cancer diagnosis. Andrea's book is a reflection of her strong belief that information is an effective weapon in the fight against cancer.

In her book "Breast Cancer Diet Cookbook For Beginners," Andrea takes readers on a journey to a world in which making educated decisions improves health results. Her dedication to nutrition based on research and her humane knowledge of the human condition make this book an invaluable tool for anybody looking for direction on the path from diagnosis to recovery.

Andrea T. Rockwell's work demonstrates her steadfast belief that a knowledgeable approach to nutrition may serve as a cornerstone for long-term health and wellbeing. Andrea expresses in her writing not just her expertise but also her sincere concern for those who set out on the road to recovery.

Table of Contents:

Introduction

While figuring out the ins and outs of a breast cancer diagnosis can be overwhelming, it's important to be proactive about your health and educate yourself on the vital role diet plays.

On these pages, we examine the studies that support the strong correlation between diet and breast cancer. This comprehensive book will empower you on your journey to recovery with its insights, practical strategies, and assortment of recipes. It does more than simply recommend foods for you to consume.

Recognizing the Dietary Effects on Breast Cancer

Research has shown that particular food choices and behaviors can significantly influence an individual's risk of developing breast cancer. We look at the impacts of various nutrients, antioxidants, and bioactive compounds found in food. Those who are aware of this connection are in a better position to make choices that might promote overall wellbeing and breast health prevention. By learning about the molecular impacts of food on the body, readers may adopt a proactive and self-reliant approach towards their nutrition.

Getting Through the First Diagnosis Process

Being told you have breast cancer is a challenging and upsetting experience. Advice on how to manage the initial days after receiving such news can be found in this section. It covers the important aspects of understanding the diagnosis process, potential treatment options, and the value of speaking with a medical professional. We discuss the emotional journey people undergo at this time in addition to the clinical aspects. This section aims to give information about coping mechanisms, support systems, and self-care so that individuals feel prepared to face a breast cancer diagnosis in its early stages with bravery and understanding.

Chapter 1

The Science Behind Nutrition and Breast Cancer

To comprehend the science underlying nutrition and its connection to breast cancer, one must investigate the complex interrelationships that exist between dietary decisions, biological mechanisms, and the onset of cancer.

- Cellular pathways that either stimulate or impede the development of breast cancer are influenced by nutrition. For example, certain nutrients and bioactive substances found in diet may alter DNA repair processes, apoptosis (programmed cell death), and cell signaling pathways.

- Oxidative stress and chronic inflammation have been linked to the development of cancer, particularly breast cancer. Foods strong in nutrients, especially those high in antioxidants like vitamins C and E, may reduce inflammation and combat oxidative stress, which may lower the risk of cancer.

- Breast cancer is significantly influenced by hormonal variables, particularly in situations where the hormone receptor is positive. Hormone levels can be influenced by nutrition; for instance, a diet high in fiber may help control estrogen levels, potentially reducing the risk of hormone-related cancers.

- Gene expression is influenced by epigenetic changes, which do not change the underlying DNA sequence. A number of nutrients, including folate and other methyl donors, may have an impact on epigenetic mechanisms and consequently alter the expression of genes linked to the development of cancer.

- Trillions of bacteria make up the gut microbiome, which has become an important factor in both health and illness. An imbalance in the microbiota has been connected to inflammation and cancer. Nutrition affects the microbiome's makeup and function.

- Insulin resistance can lead to chronic inflammation and may be a factor in the development of breast cancer. It is frequently linked to diets high in processed foods and refined sugars. The best insulin sensitivity is supported by a healthy weight and a balanced diet.

- Certain nutrients show signs of being anti-cancer. Cruciferous vegetables, for example, provide substances like sulforaphane that may offer some cancer-prevention benefits. Fatty fish, which are high in omega-3 fatty acids, have anti-inflammatory qualities.

Beyond specific nutritional requirements, lifestyle choices like eating a healthy weight and getting regular exercise improve general well being and may also have an indirect impact on the risk of breast cancer.

Plant-based diets like the Mediterranean diet, for example, have an emphasis on a range of whole foods that have anti-cancer qualities. These dietary patterns offer a comprehensive approach to nutrition by including fruits, vegetables, whole grains, and healthy fats.

Overview of Breast Cancer

Breast cancer is a complicated and common type of cancer that starts in the breast tissue's cells. Although it may happen to males as well as women, it affects women much more frequently. Comprehending the fundamental elements of breast cancer is imperative for prompt identification, management, and general well-being.

1. Breast cancer types:
Breast cancer is a multifactorial illness with different etiologies, growth patterns, and clinical features. Breast cancers can be classified into two main categories: non-invasive (in situ) and invasive, including subtypes such as invasive ductal carcinoma (IDC) and ductal carcinoma in situ (DCIS).

2. Risk variables:
The chance of getting breast cancer is influenced by a variety of variables. These include genetic mutations (BRCA1 and BRCA2), age, gender, and family history. Hormonal factors (early menstruation, late menopause, hormone replacement therapy), and lifestyle factors (diet, physical activity, alcohol consumption).

3. Prompt Identification and Evaluation:

Treatment results are considerably improved by early identification. Finding anomalies requires the use of mammography, clinical breast exams, and breast self-examinations. It is advised that people have regular tests, particularly if they have risk factors or a family history of breast cancer.

4. Symptoms:

Breast cancer symptoms can vary, but they may include thickening or lumping of the breast, changes in breast size or form, skin abnormalities (dimpling, redness), abnormalities in the nipples, and unexplained breast discomfort. Healthcare practitioners should be informed of any worrying developments as soon as possible.

5. Diagnosis:

To ascertain the kind and stage of the cancer, the diagnosis combines tissue biopsy with imaging tests including mammography and ultrasound. Depending on each instance, more testing—including genetic testing—might be advised.

6. Staging:

Treatment options are guided by staging, which establishes the amount of cancer dissemination. Breast cancer is generally staged using the TNM method (tumor size, lymph node involvement, metastasis), which goes from Stage 0 (in situ) to Stage IV (advanced, metastatic cancer).

7. Treatment Modalities:

Treatment for breast cancer is tailored according to the kind, stage, and condition of the patient. Radiation treatment, chemotherapy, hormone therapy, targeted therapy, immunotherapy, and surgery (mastectomy or lumpectomy) are common techniques. Plans for treatment could combine these strategies.

8. Afterlife and Repercussions: Survival rates have increased dramatically as a result of developments in breast cancer research and therapy. Following initial treatment, patients go onto the survivorship phase, which entails routine follow-up appointments, recurrence monitoring, and discussion of any possible long-term therapeutic side effects.

9. Assistive Healthcare:
Breast cancer presents both physical and emotional issues that need supportive treatment. Individuals' general well-being is enhanced by support groups, psychotherapy, and holistic approaches to care throughout their cancer experience.

Link between Diet and Cancer

A great deal of study has been done on the complex and dynamic interaction between nutrition and cancer. There is no one meal that may prevent or treat cancer, but a growing body of research indicates that dietary decisions have a significant impact on cancer risk.

Carcinogenic Compounds Substances that have the potential to cause cancer are known as carcinogens, and some dietary components may include them. For example, eating meat that has been grilled or scorched at a high temperature can create compounds called polycyclic aromatic hydrocarbons (PAHs) and heterocyclic amines (HCAs), which are linked to a higher risk of developing certain types of cancer.

Phytochemicals and Antioxidants Antioxidants and phytochemicals, found in abundance in fruits, vegetables, whole grains, and legumes, offer protection against cancer. Free radicals are unstable chemicals that may damage DNA, and these substances aid in the neutralization of cancer development.

Connecting Inflammation with Cancer

Numerous malignancies are known to be influenced by chronic inflammation. Diets high in sugar, processed foods, and saturated fats may be a factor in the development of systemic inflammation. On the other hand, foods high in anti-inflammatory compounds, as those in a Mediterranean diet, could be beneficial.

Insulin Resistance and Cancer

Diets heavy in foods with a high glycemic index that raise blood sugar quickly may be linked to insulin resistance. Increased amounts of insulin and insulin-like growth factor (IGF), which can encourage cell proliferation and perhaps play a role in the development of cancer, are linked to insulin resistance.

Cancer Risk with Obesity

One known risk factor for several malignancies is obesity. Diets heavy in foods rich in calories but low in nutrients can cause obesity and weight gain. Hormones and growth are produced by adipose tissue that may influence cancer development.

The influence of hormones

Breast and ovarian cancers are examples of hormone receptor-positive malignancies, which are largely influenced by hormones, especially estrogen. Hormone levels may be impacted by specific diets. Phytoestrogens, for instance, are found in soy products and may have both estrogenic and anti-estrogenic properties.

Dietary fiber and digestive cancers

Fruits, vegetables, and whole grains are high in dietary fiber, which has been linked to a decreased risk of colorectal and other digestive cancers. In addition to encouraging regular bowel movements, fiber may aid in the removal of certain carcinogens from the digestive system.

Alcohol and Cancer

Drinking alcohol has been associated with a higher risk of developing breast, liver, and colorectal cancers, among other cancers. The processes include the influence on hormone levels and the transformation of alcohol into the recognized carcinogen acetaldehyde.

Nutritionally Balanced Diet for Cancer Prevention

It's important to prevent cancer by eating a diet rich in a range of nutrient-dense foods. A variety of protective chemicals may be obtained from a plant-based diet that includes a wide variety of fruits, vegetables, whole grains, lean meats, and healthy fats.

Individual Variability

It's critical to understand that every person reacts differently to dietary components. A person's lifestyle, general health, and genetic makeup all influence how nutrition and cancer risk interact.

Key Nutrients and Their Role in Cancer Prevention:

Cancer can be prevented in large part via nutrition, and some nutrients have been shown to reduce the chance of developing the disease.

1. Antioxidants (selenium, vitamins C and E):

Free radicals are unstable chemicals that can damage DNA and aid in the development of cancer. Antioxidants neutralize these molecules. Selenium, along with vitamins C and E, functions as a potent antioxidant that shields cells from oxidative damage.

2. Vitamin D:

Vitamin D has been associated with a lower risk of some malignancies, such as colorectal, prostate, and breast cancer, and is essential for keeping strong bones. It aids in immune system and cell development control.

3. Fatty Acids Omega-3:

Omega-3 fatty acids, which are present in walnuts, flaxseeds, and fatty fish (such as salmon and mackerel), have anti-inflammatory qualities. Prolonged inflammation is linked with cancer development, and incorporating omega-3s may help mitigate this risk.

4. Folate:
Vitamin B plays a crucial role in the creation and repair of DNA. Folate-rich diets, which are found in leafy greens, legumes, and fortified grains, may help lower the risk of malignancies like colon cancer that involve fast cell division.

5. Calcium:
Not only is calcium essential for healthy bones, but it may also help prevent colon cancer. Good sources of calcium include dairy products, leafy greens, and fortified plant-based milk.

6. Fiber:
Diets rich in fiber, which is present in whole grains, fruits, and vegetables, support healthy digestion and may reduce the risk of colorectal cancer. Fiber promotes regular bowel movements, which assist the digestive tract rid itself of any carcinogens.

7.   Phytochemicals: Carotenoids   and Flavonoids:
Phytochemicals are substances that might potentially prevent cancer and are present in a wide range of fruits and vegetables. For example, flavonoids and carotenoids have anti-inflammatory   and   antioxidant properties.

8. Cruciferous vegetables, (such as Brussels sprouts and broccoli):
Sulforaphane, one of the chemicals in these veggies, has been shown to have anti-cancer capabilities. Regular intake may be linked to a decreased chance of developing some malignancies, such as prostate and breast cancer, according to studies.

9. Epigallocatechin Gallate, or EGCG, Green Tea:
Green tea has antioxidant-rich polyphenols, including EGCG. Frequent intake may help lower the risk of cancer, since studies have

suggested that it may have preventive benefits against a number of malignancies.

10. Curcumin:
The main ingredient of Turmeric, plays an anti-inflammatory and antioxidant role in the plant. It may be able to prevent cancer, according to research, especially if it slows down the proliferation of cancer cells.

11. Zinc:
Zinc aids in DNA repair and immune system function. Consuming enough zinc, which is included in foods like meat, nuts, and seeds, promotes general health and may help prevent cancer.

12. Beta-Carotene:
Beta-carotene, a precursor of vitamin A, is present in orange and yellow foods. It has antioxidant properties and may offer protection against some malignancies, especially non-smoker lung cancer.

Chapter 2

Developing a Healthy Eating Plan

Establishing a nutritious diet is essential to general health and can play a big role in managing and preventing a number of diseases, including cancer.

Basics of a Balanced Diet:

Portion Control: Control your serving sizes to prevent overindulging. Pay attention to your body's signals of hunger and fullness and be cautious of portion amounts. A balanced diet gives you energy that lasts all day.

Lean Proteins: Include low-fat dairy, fish, chicken, beans, lentils, and tofu as well as other lean protein sources. Immune system performance, muscle repair, and general cellular health all depend on proteins.

Whole Grains: For more fiber, vitamins, and minerals, opt for whole grains rather than processed grains. Brown rice, quinoa, whole wheat, oats, and barley are a few examples.

Healthy Fat: Consume foods high in unsaturated fats, such as olive oil, avocados, almonds, and seeds. These fats are necessary for the brain, the body's general cardiovascular health, and the absorption of nutrients.

Colorful Fruits and Vegetables: When creating your meal, try to include a range of fruits and vegetables. Variations in hue denote distinct nutritional profiles that offer a multitude of vitamins, minerals, and antioxidants.

Dairy or Dairy Alternatives: Eat dairy or dairy substitutes that have been fortified to provide vitamin D and calcium. The health of your bones depends on these nutrients. Yogurt, milk, and fortified plant-based milk are among the options.

Tailoring Nutrition to Individual Needs

Age, gender, exercise level, health issues, and personal objectives are some of the variables that affect an individual's nutritional needs.

Calorie Needs: Recognize your personal calorie requirements depending on your age, height, weight, degree of exercise, and general health objectives. This guarantees a sufficient energy intake without consuming too many calories.

Macro Function Ratios: Modify the proportions of proteins, fats, and carbs in accordance with your personal health objectives. A balanced distribution may be beneficial for people trying to control their weight, while athletes may need to consume more protein.

Dietary limits: Take into account any dietary choices or limits, including veganism, vegetarianism, and some food allergies. A well-chosen diet plan should fulfill nutritional requirements without leading to deficits.

Medical illnesses: When managing medical illnesses, take into account particular dietary recommendations. For instance, those with diabetes might need to watch how much carbohydrates they eat, whereas others with cardiovascular problems would want to concentrate on heart-healthy fats.

Hydration Needs: Taking into account individual aspects such as climate, level of physical activity, and general health, appropriately attend to hydration needs. Digestion, nutrition absorption, temperature control, and general physiological processes all depend on water.

Importance of Adequate Hydration:

Staying well hydrated is essential to preserving your best health and wellbeing.

Transport of nutrients, the removal of waste, and general cellular function all depend on water. It aids in the body's production of energy and preservation of equilibrium.

By encouraging the breakdown and absorption of nutrients, hydration facilitates digestion. It promotes general gastrointestinal health and aids in the prevention of constipation.

The body naturally cools itself by sweating. Drinking plenty of water aids in controlling body temperature, particularly in hot climates and when engaging in physical exercise.

By lubricating and cushioning the joints, adequate hydration promotes joint health. This is especially crucial for people who participate in physically demanding activities that strain their joints.

Dehydration can have a detrimental effect on cognitive function, resulting in tiredness, trouble focusing, and memory loss. Maintaining proper hydration promotes brain health.

Drinking enough water is essential for getting the most out of your workouts. Physical stamina, strength, and general sports performance can all be negatively impacted by even minor dehydration.

Staying hydrated is important for preserving the suppleness of the skin and avoiding dryness. A balanced water consumption promotes general skin health and a good complexion.

Through urine, water aids in the body's removal of waste and poisons. Kidney function and general detoxification depend on this.

Chapter 3

Nutritional Strategies during Treatment

Addressing Nutrient Needs during Therapy:

Cancer treatment may put the body through a lot, which can have an impact on nutrition and general health. Maintaining strength, controlling side effects, and assisting the body's coping mechanisms during treatments all depend on attending to nutritional demands.

A comprehensive evaluation by a licensed dietician or other medical expert should come first. Think about the kind of cancer, the available treatment options, your present nutritional state, and any underlying medical issues. Customized plans take special demands into consideration and assist in adjusting techniques as necessary.

Keep an eye on your calorie intake to avoid unintentional weight loss. Energy needs may rise as a result of cancer and its therapies. Modify the meal schedule, include nutrient-dense snacks, and adjust portion sizes to control treatment-related symptoms while maintaining an adequate energy intake.

Protein is essential for immunological response, tissue healing, and muscular mass maintenance. Make foods high in protein, such lean meats, poultry, fish, eggs, dairy, legumes, and tofu, a priority. Based on adverse effects from medication that may affect appetite, modify protein intake.

Keep an eye on your hydration, particularly when receiving therapies that might lead to fluid retention or dehydration. Sufficient fluid intake promotes general health, aids in the management of adverse consequences including constipation, and maintains renal function. Adapt your fluid intake to your unique needs and the demands of your treatment.

To supply the body with vital vitamins and minerals, prioritize consuming meals that are high in nutrients. A range of vibrant fruits, vegetables, entire grains, and healthy fats should be included. Foods high in nutrients help the body get the vital nutrients it needs to repair.

If side effects from medication cause you to miss meals, think about taking nutritional supplements. Multivitamins, minerals, or certain nutrients that medical practitioners suggest are examples of supplements. To prevent potential interactions, dietary supplements should be customized to each patient's needs and monitored closely by medical professionals.

During cancer therapy, nausea and taste alterations are typical. Choose simple or cold dishes, use new cooking techniques, and drink plenty of water. You can control nausea by eating small, frequent meals and snacks. Work together with a dietician to develop individualized approaches for dealing with taste changes.

Incorporate meals high in fiber to maintain digestive health, taking into account any gastrointestinal complaints. To encourage regular bowel movements, gradually introduce high-fiber meals such as fruits, vegetables, and whole grains. Consuming enough fiber helps avoid constipation, which is a typical adverse reaction to several medications.

Respond proactively to weight fluctuations in light of treatment outcomes. Increase your protein and calorie intake if you're losing weight unintentionally. Give lower-calorie, higher-nutrient products priority if you're worried about gaining weight. Effective management of weight swings is aided by routine monitoring.

Keep lines of communication open with the experts on the healthcare team, such as nutritionists, oncologists, and others. For best results, regular follow-ups and dietary plan modifications based on treatment responses and evolving needs are essential.

Use dietary techniques to combat weariness. Make energy-boosting foods your first priority, drink plenty of water, and think about introducing smaller, more frequent meals. Sufficient diet promotes general energy levels and aids in the management of weariness.

Adjust cooking techniques and meal planning according to personal tastes and adverse reactions. To adapt to shifting tastes, try experimenting with various flavors, textures, and temperatures. Make meal preparation simpler during periods of fatigue or low energy.

Combat Common Side Effects Through Diet

Making wise food decisions is essential to preventing frequent adverse effects of cancer therapy, preserving nutritional status, improving wellbeing, and bolstering the body's resistance. This is a thorough dietary advice to help counter frequent side effects:

Nausea and Vomiting
Foods to Combat:

- Ginger: Used as a spice, in tea, or in soups, ginger is well-known for its anti-nausea qualities.

- Peppermint: Candies or tea with peppermint extract may assist with nausea.

- Bland meals: Opt for simple, quickly digested meals like bread, rice, or crackers.

Hydration Tip: Drink clear, cold liquids throughout the day, such as water, ginger ale, or herbal teas, to stay hydrated.

Taste-Change
Food To Combat:

- Choose meals with strong tastes, including onions, garlic, or spicy spices.

- Citrus Fruits: Refreshing flavors may be found in tangy fruits like oranges and grapefruits.

- Cold Foods: You could find it easier to enjoy cold foods or drinks.

Hydration Tip: For a tasty twist, add cucumber or citrus fruit slices to water.

Appetite Loss
Foods to combat:

- Nutrient-Dense Smoothies:Combine yogurt, fruits, veggies, and protein powder to make a filling beverage.

- Small, Frequent Meals: Rather than three large meals a day, choose to eat smaller, more frequent ones.

- Favorite meals: To stimulate appetite, include meals that you are acquainted with and enjoy.

Hydration Tip: Drink hydrating drinks, such as smoothies or diluted fruit juices, in between meals to stay hydrated.

Fatigue
Foods to Fight:

- Complex Carbohydrates: Legumes, whole grains, and starchy vegetables all offer long-lasting energy.

- Snacks High in Protein: Cheese, yogurt, nuts, and seeds can all help sustain energy levels.

Hydration Tips: Make sure you're getting enough fluids in because dehydration might make you feel tired.

Drinking plenty of water with a squeeze of citrus or herbal teas may be hydrating and refreshing.

Diarrhea:
Foods to Combat:

- Bananas: High in potassium and easily digested.

- White rice: Easy on the digestive tract and helpful in bulking up stool.

- Boiled potatoes: Give you energy without making your diarrhea worse.

Hydration Tip: Rehydrate with electrolyte-rich liquids, such as coconut water or sports drinks.

Constipation
Foods to Combat:

- Foods High in Fiber: These consist of whole grains, legumes, fruits, and vegetables.

- Prunes or Prune Juice: These inherently laxative foods can help facilitate bowel motions.

Hydration Tips: Drink plenty of water to help loosen stools.

- Mild laxative effects may be caused by warm liquids, such as herbal teas.

Dry Mouth and Difficulty Swallowing. Foods to Combat:

- Foods That Swell: To increase moisture content, choose soups, stews, or foods that have sauces.

- Hydrating Fruits: Fruits high in water content, such as oranges or watermelon, might help relieve dry mouth.

- Sugar-Free Candy or Gum: Promotes the production of saliva.

Hydration Tips: Drink water throughout the day to stay hydrated, and use a straw to make it simpler.

.

Changes in Weight
Foods to Combat:

- High-Calorie Snacks: Granola, cheese, nuts, and butter may all add calories to a snack.

- Protein-Rich Foods: Lean proteins such as fish, fowl, and tofu help maintain muscle mass.

- Nutrient-Dense Meals: For general health, prioritize eating balanced, nutrient-rich meals.

Hydration Tip: Caloric drinks that are high in calories, such as shakes or smoothies, can help you maintain your weight.

Dehydration
Foods to Combat:

- Foods That Rehydrate: fruits and vegetables high in water content, such as celery, cucumbers, and watermelon.

- Soups and Broths: Offer vital nutrients and water.

- Herbal teas: Provide taste and hydration.
Hydration Tip: Plan to take regular breaks during the day to sip water.

Malnutrition
Foods to Combat:
- Balanced Meals: For complete nutrition, give priority to a range of nutrient-dense meals.

- Fortified Foods: Select goods that have been fortified with minerals and vitamins.

- Protein Supplements: As directed by medical specialists, including smoothies or bars high in protein.

Hydration Tips: Drink nutrient-rich liquids, such as fortified plant-based milks or vegetable juices, as a hydration tip.

Collaboration with Healthcare Team
- Consult medical specialists on a regular basis, such as nutritionists and oncologists.

- Provide updates on dietary modifications, personal preferences, and any lingering adverse effects.

- Work together to modify dietary plans in response to each person's unique experience.

Chapter 4

Functional and Dysfunctional Foods

Exploring Foods with Health-Boosting Properties

Functional foods provide extra health advantages over and above basic nutrition, which can enhance general wellbeing. By including certain items in your diet, you can extend your life, support certain physiological processes, and help avoid disease.

Berries
Health Benefits:
- Abundant antioxidants, which aid in preventing oxidative stress.
- Anti-inflammatory qualities could be beneficial to cardiac health.

- A high fiber diet promotes weight control and intestinal health.

Fatty Fish (Salmon, Mackerel, Sardines)
Health Benefits:
- Omega-3 fatty acids are vital for brain function and cognitive health.
- They lower inflammation and promote heart health.
- Could help lower the chance of developing chronic illnesses.

Leafy Greens (Kale, Spinach, Swiss Chard)
Health Benefits:
- Rich in minerals, vitamins, and antioxidants.
- High in fiber, which supports both weight control and digestive health.
- Anti-inflammatory qualities promote general health.

Turmeric
Health Benefits:
- Has curcumin, which has strong anti-inflammatory properties.
- May lower the chance of developing chronic illnesses.
- Promotes joint health and could be advantageous for cognition.

Yogurt (Probiotic-Rich)
Health Benefits:
- Offers healthy probiotics to support intestinal health.
- Packed with vital minerals, calcium, and protein; may support a strong immune system.

Nuts and Seeds (Almonds, Walnuts, Chia Seeds)
Health Benefits:
-Great sources of heart-healthy fats that promote cardiac health Packed with minerals, vitamins, and antioxidants.

- Nuts and seeds might help you control your weight.

Garlic
Health Benefits:
- Has allicin, which is well-known for its antibacterial qualities.
- May improve heart health and decrease blood pressure.
- Anti-inflammatory properties improve health in general.

Green Tea
Health Benefits:
- High in antioxidants, especially catechins; may help maintain a healthy metabolism and help control body weight.
- Has substances that may be able to combat cancer.

Quinoa
Health Benefits:
- Excellent source of protein that is good for vegans.

- High in fiber, which supports satiety and digestive health.
- Offers vital minerals and vitamins.

Sweet Potatoes
Health Benefits:
- Abundant in vitamins, particularly beta-carotene, which is a precursor of vitamin A.
- Rich in fiber, which promotes intestinal well-being.
- Could aid in controlling blood sugar levels.

Identifying Foods to Limit or Avoid:

It's important to identify and limit or avoid specific foods that may contribute to health difficulties while creating a balanced diet, in addition to focusing on including functional foods that give health advantages. This methodology guarantees a thorough and balanced dietary regimen.

Processed Meats (Limit):
 Concerns:

-       Rich in salt and saturated fats; associated with a higher risk of heart disease and several types of cancer.
- The balanced diet approach is to pick lean protein sources such as fish, poultry, and plant-based proteins and to limit intake.

Sugary Beverages (Avoid/Limit):
 Concerns:

-Rich in added sugars, which raises the risk of type 2 diabetes and dental problems while also causing weight gain and obesity.
- Well-Rounded Diet Method: - As alternatives, choose for water, herbal teas, or unsweetened drinks. Consume in moderation if you do.

Fast Food (Limit):
 Concerns:

- Usually heavy in salt and harmful trans fats; frequent intake is associated with metabolic problems, obesity, and heart disease.

- Balanced Diet Approach: - Make homemade meals with fresh ingredients a priority and save fast food for special occasions.

Processed Snacks (Limit):
Concerns:

- frequently include high concentrations of harmful fats and processed sugars.

Low in vital nutrients, which increases the consumption of empty calories.

- Balanced Diet Approach: - Select whole, less processed snacks for optimal nutritional density, such as fruits, nuts, or yogurt.

Sugar-Sweetened Cereals (Limit/Avoid):
Concerns:

- High in added sugars, particularly seen in well-known breakfast cereals; linked to a higher risk of obesity and metabolic problems.

- Balanced Diet Approach: - Give whole foods or low-sugar cereals preference for breakfast.

Deep-Fried Foods (Limit):
Concerns:

- Rich in harmful trans and saturated fats; frequent intake is associated with weight gain and cardiovascular illnesses.

- Balanced Diet Approach: - Prefer baking, grilling, or sautéing over deep-frying as your cooking methods.

Highly Processed Foods (Limit):
Concerns:

- frequently have too much salt, preservatives, and additives.

Absence of vital nutrients included in whole, unprocessed diets.

- Balanced Diet Approach: - To regulate ingredients and nutrient content, prioritize whole foods and make meals at home.

Artificially Sweetened Foods (Limit):
Concerns:

- May interfere with gut microbiota and metabolic functions.

- The effects of artificial sweeteners on long-term health are currently being studied.

- The balanced diet approach is to use natural sweeteners sparingly, such as honey or maple syrup, and to watch how much artificial sweeteners you consume.

White Bread and Refined Grains (Limit):
Concerns:

- Absence of vital minerals and fiber present in whole grains.

- Quickly increase blood sugar levels, which may lead to insulin resistance.

- Balanced Diet Approach: - For higher nutritional content, use whole grains such brown rice, quinoa, and whole wheat bread.

Highly Salted Foods (Limit):
  Concerns:

- Overconsumption of salt is associated with cardiovascular disease and hypertension.

- Encourage water retention and possible renal problems.

- The balanced diet approach is to flavor food with herbs and spices rather than a lot of salt. When low-sodium options are available, pick them.

Building a Balanced Diet with Functional Foods:

1. Use an Assortment of Fruits and Vegetables:

- To guarantee a wide variety of vitamins, minerals, and antioxidants, aim for a rainbow of hues.

2. Select Whole Grains:

- To increase dietary fiber and nutrient intake, choose whole grains such as brown rice, quinoa, oats, and whole wheat.

3. Make Lean Proteins a Priority:
- To maintain muscular health, include lean protein sources such as fish, chicken, lentils, and plant-based proteins.

4. Incorporate Healthy Fats:
- For heart health and satiety, include sources of healthy fats such avocados, nuts, seeds, and olive oil.

5. Accept Foods High in Probiotics:
    - Include kefir, sauerkraut, kimchi, or yogurt to enhance immune system function and gastrointestinal health.

6. Mindful Portion Control:
- Keep an eye on portion sizes to keep your energy intake and expenditure in check.

7. Stay Hydrated:Make drinking water a priority throughout the day, and cut out on sugary or calorically-rich drinks.

8. Cook at Home: - To have control over ingredients, cooking techniques, and total nutrient content, prepare meals at home.

9. Limit Added Sugars: Choose natural sweeteners instead of added sugars found in processed meals.

10. Frequent Physical Activity: To enhance general health and wellbeing, combine a balanced diet with frequent physical activity.

Chapter 5

Anti-Cancer Diets

Overview of Anti-Cancer Diets

By highlighting nutrient-rich foods and lifestyle choices, anti-cancer diets seek to both improve overall health and lower the chance of developing cancer. Plant-based diets and the Mediterranean diet are two well-known anti-cancer dietary strategies.

1. **Mediterranean Diet:**

   - Ample amounts of legumes, whole grains, fruits, and veggies.

   - A focus on omega-3 fatty acids from fish and olive oil.

   - Moderate intake of chicken, dairy products, and red wine.

   - Minimal consumption of prepared meals and red meat.

Rationale
- High in fiber, omega-3 fatty acids, and antioxidants.
- May lessen inflammation and promote general health.
- Associated with a decreased risk of several malignancies, including colorectal and breast cancers.

2. **Plant-Based Diet:**
- Mostly consists of foods that are derived from plants, including whole grains, fruits, vegetables, nuts, and seeds.
- Minimal or nonexistent animal products, such as dairy and meat.
- A focus on a variety of vibrant plant meals in order to optimize nutritional intake.

Rationale:
- Rich in phytochemicals, vitamins, minerals, and fiber.
- Plant components may have anti-inflammatory and anti-cancer effects.

- Linked to a lower risk of many malignancies, including prostate and breast cancer.

Research Supporting Anti-Cancer Diet Approaches:

Adopting the principles of an anti-cancer diet is strongly supported by nutritional studies and research. Important discoveries demonstrate how these diets may lower cancer risk and improve general health.

1. Inflammation Reduction: Plant-based and Mediterranean diets have been linked to anti-inflammatory properties that may reduce the risk of cancer and other chronic illnesses.

2. Antioxidant Protection:
Both strategies emphasize diets high in fruits and vegetables, which are rich in

antioxidants that help fend off free radicals and shield cells from harm.

3. Weight Control:

Retaining a healthy weight is essential to preventing cancer. Anti-cancer diets help with weight management since they emphasize complete, nutrient-dense meals.

4. Balanced Macronutrients:

These diets support a macronutrient balance by placing an emphasis on lean proteins, complex carbs, and healthy fats. This promotes general wellbeing.

5. Gut Microbiota Health:

A varied and healthy gut microbiota is particularly supported by plant-based diets and is involved in immune response and inflammatory management.

6. Decreased Intake of Processed Foods:

Red and processed meats have been connected to an elevated risk of various malignancies, hence both diets forbid their consumption.

7. Cardiovascular Health: -
 Because the Mediterranean diet lowers the risk of cardiovascular disorders, it indirectly helps prevent cancer. This is because it contains heart-healthy ingredients.

8. Hormonal Balance:
Plant-based diets may have an impact on hormonal balance, particularly with regard to estrogen levels, which may lower the risk of malignancies linked to hormones.

Foods That Fight Cancer

Overview of Anti-Cancer Foods:

- Colorful Fruits and Vegetables:
- Berries: Antioxidants that fight oxidative stress are abundant in blueberries, strawberries, and raspberries.

- Leafy Greens: Rich in vitamins, minerals, and phytochemicals include spinach, kale, and Swiss chard.

- Cruciferous Vegetables: Sulforaphane, which has been linked to possible anti-cancer effects, is present in broccoli, cauliflower, and Brussels sprouts.

- **Turmeric:**

- contains curcumin, an antioxidant and effective anti-inflammatory substance that may be able to prevent cancer..

- **Garlic:**

- Garlic, which is high in allicin, has been found to have anti-cancer properties and may help lower the chance of developing some cancers.

- **Ginger:**

- has antioxidant and anti-inflammatory qualities, which may have an impact on cancer prevention.

- Tomatoes:
- Include lycopene, an antioxidant linked to a decreased risk of some cancers, such as prostate and breast cancers.

- Green tea:
- Green tea, which is high in catechins, may offer protection against certain cancer types.

- Nuts and Seeds:
- Rich sources of antioxidants, fiber, and healthy fats may be found in almonds, walnuts, chia seeds, and flax seeds.

- Fatty Fish:
Omega-3 fatty acids, which have anti-inflammatory qualities, are abundant in salmon, mackerel, and sardines.

- Legumes:
- Chickpeas, lentils, and beans are a great source of protein, fiber, and other nutrients.

- Whole Grains:

Oats, brown rice, quinoa, and whole wheat all add important minerals and fiber to a diet.

Incorporating Superfoods into Daily Meals:

Recipes for Smoothie and meal ideas

It is possible to incorporate anti-cancer foods into your everyday meals in a tasty and nourishing way.

1. Smoothie Bowl with Berries:

Yogurt Parfait with Berries. Combine mixed berries with plant-based yogurt or another dairy substitute to create a vibrant and high-in antioxidant smoothie bowl. Add some nuts and seeds on top for some extra nutrition and texture.

2. Turmeric Golden Milk:

- Blend turmeric, plant-based milk, a tiny bit of black pepper, and a tiny bit of sweetness to make a comforting turmeric golden milk. Savor it as a calming beverage.

3. Tomato and Avocado Salad:

This light salad full of beneficial fats and lycopene is made by combining tomatoes, avocados, and leafy greens.

4. Quinoa with Green Tea Infusion:

This adaptable whole grain may get a mild taste and possible health advantages by cooking it with green tea.

5. Seeds and Nuts Trail Mix:

- Combine a range of nuts and seeds to make a trail mix. For sweetness and additional antioxidants, add dried fruits.

6. Chickpea Hummus Wrap:

- Prepare a whole-grain wrap stuffed with a mix of vibrant veggies, homemade hummus, and chickpeas.

7. Turmeric-Ginger Smoothie:

For a colorful and anti-inflammatory smoothie, blend almond milk with banana, pineapple, spinach, ginger, and a little amount of turmeric.

8. Quinoa Salad with Berries:

- For a hydrating and nutrient-dense salad, combine cooked quinoa with chopped mint, mixed berries, and a light vinaigrette.

9. Leafy Green Salad with Nuts:

For a nutrient-dense salad, mix spinach, kale, and arugula with a choice of nuts, seeds, and a light vinaigrette.

10. Mango-Green Tea Smoothie:

This nutrient-dense and delightful smoothie is made by blending mango, spinach, green tea, and a scoop of Greek yogurt.

11. Chia Seed Pudding with Berries:

To make a tasty and antioxidant-rich pudding, combine chia seeds, almond milk, a little honey, and mixed berries on top.

12. Green Tea Chia Pudding:

By combining chia seeds with plant-based milk, a little honey, and green tea. For a chia pudding that is full of nutrients and antioxidants, leave it to sit overnight.

13. Quinoa salad with three berries:

- Mix raspberries, blueberries, and strawberries with cooked quinoa. For a colorful salad, toss in some feta cheese, fresh mint, and a mild balsamic dressing.

14. Baked fish with Lemon:

- Before baking, season fish with ginger, garlic, and turmeric. Add some freshly squeezed lemon on top for a tasty and nutritious dinner.

15. Turmeric-Ginger Chicken Skewers:

To make tasty and anti-inflammatory skewers, marinate chicken pieces in a mixture of olive oil, turmeric, ginger, and garlic before grilling.

16. Garlic-Roasted Brussels Sprouts:

To make a tasty side dish, toss halved Brussels sprouts with minced garlic, olive oil, and a dash of sea salt. Roast.

17. Nutty Broccoli Quinoa Bowl:

- Transfer cooked quinoa, roasted broccoli, and a sprinkling of walnuts and almonds into a bowl.. Drizzle with a lemon-turmeric dressing.

18. Lentil and Vegetable Curry:

- With lentils, tomatoes, spinach, and a mixture of anti-inflammatory spices like cumin and turmeric, make a filling curry.

19. Broccoli with Garlic Roasted:

- Before roasting, toss broccoli florets with olive oil, chopped garlic, and a pinch of turmeric for a tasty and nutritious side dish.

20. Salmon and Avocado Sushi Bowl:

Assemble cooked brown rice, salmon, avocado slices, and seaweed strips into a deconstructed sushi bowl. Pour in some soy-ginger dressing.

21. Spiced Chickpea and Spinach Curry:

- Make a filling curry with tomatoes, spinach, and chickpeas along with a mixture of anti-inflammatory spices including ginger and turmeric.

22. Walnut-Crusted Baked Fish:

- For a crispy and omega-3-rich main dish, coat fish filets with crushed walnuts, garlic powder, and lemon zest before baking.

23. Turmeric-Spiced Vegetable Stir-Fry:

For a vibrant and anti-inflammatory dinner, combine broccoli, bell peppers, and tofu with a stir-fry sauce flavored with turmeric.

24. Garlic and Ginger Stir-Fry:

To make a tasty and nutrient-rich dinner, stir-fry some vegetables with garlic and ginger. For even more anti-cancer effects, including cruciferous veggies like broccoli in your diet.

Chapter 6

Maintaining a Healthy Weight

Balancing Nutrition and Weight Management:

1. Foods High in Vitamins, Minerals, and Essential Nutrients:
   - Give priority to foods high in these nutrients.
   - Vary your intake of whole grains, fruits, vegetables, lean meats, and healthy fats.

2. Portion Control:
   - To avoid overindulging, pay attention to portion proportions.
   - To improve mindful eating, use smaller plates, pay attention to hunger cues, and enjoy every meal.

3. Hydration:
 - Drink water to keep hydrated throughout the day. - As thirst and hunger may often be confused, maintaining enough hydration will help reduce needless eating.

4. Balanced Macronutrients:
 - Make sure that every meal has an equal amount of lipids, proteins, and carbs.
 - Make healthy fats, lean proteins, and complex carbs your top priorities for long-lasting energy and fullness.

5. Frequent Physical Activity:
 - Including cardiovascular, strength, and flexibility workouts in your routine can help you control your weight and improve your general health.

6. Mindful Eating:
 - Eat mindfully, observing your hunger and fullness cues.
 - Reduce outside distractions when eating, and enjoy the tastes of every bite.

7. A Focus on whole Foods:
- Opt for entire, less processed foods rather than highly processed and refined ones.
- In addition to offering vital nutrients, whole meals frequently include more fiber, which increases feelings of fullness.

8. Consistency and Sustainability:
- Make long-term, sustainable dietary adjustments.
- Long-term, consistent healthy eating practices are more beneficial than temporary, restricted ones.

9. Seek Professional Advice:
- For individualized advice, speak with a registered dietitian or other healthcare provider.
- Experts may assist in customizing diet regimens to meet each person's needs, taking into account aspects like age, gender, and medical concerns.

Strategies for Weight Control during Treatment:

Work with medical experts to create plans for individualized nutrition.
Customize dietary plans to meet the nutritional requirements and negative effects of certain treatments.

Eat smaller, more regular meals over the day. This strategy can assist in controlling hunger and halting weight loss while undergoing therapy.

To assist muscular maintenance, give priority to meals high in protein.
Fish, poultry, lentils, dairy products, and lean meats can all help you get enough protein.

Talk to medical specialists about whether you might need to take nutrient supplements.

During therapy, supplements can fill in nutritional shortages and guarantee that vital vitamins and minerals are preserved.

Monitor calorie intake without going overboard. During therapy, having enough energy is critical. It's important to balance nutrient-dense meals with calorie requirements.

Modify physical activity in accordance with energy levels and side effects of medication. Include mild workouts like yoga or strolling, adjusting the intensity as necessary.

Take care of side symptoms including nausea or taste alterations that might affect nutrition.
Collaborate with medical specialists to identify remedies, such as dietary or medication changes

During therapy, look for psychosocial assistance to help you deal with emotional difficulties.
Maintaining a healthy weight is facilitated by a supportive environment, because emotional and physical health are intertwined.

Keep a close eye on your weight, nutritional health, and side effects from therapy.
Modify diet regimens as necessary to ensure continued assistance and flexibility in response to evolving situations.

Chapter 7

Mindful Eating for Emotional Well-being

Coping with Emotional Challenges:

Understanding Emotional Triggers

Acknowledge the emotions that impact one's eating patterns. Fostering a mindful approach to emotional well-being begins with an understanding of the relationship between emotions and eating.

Embracing Emotional Resilience

Develop emotional resilience by engaging in exercises like yoga, deep breathing, or mindfulness meditation.

Developing emotional resilience makes it easier to deal with emotional difficulties without turning just to food for solace.

Journaling for Self-Reflection

Monitor trends in your eating and emotional intake by keeping a journal.

It is possible to make good behavioral adjustments and get useful insights into eating patterns by reflecting on emotional states and their accompanying eating habits.

Seeking Professional Assistance

Seek advice from mental health specialists. - Counselors or therapists with training can offer strategies for overcoming emotional obstacles and creating a better connection with food.

Mindful Eating Techniques:

1. Savoring Every Bite:
- Take your time eating so you may properly enjoy the tastes, textures, and scents.
- Incorporating all of your senses into your dining experience increases enjoyment and lowers the risk of overindulging.

2. Mindful Meal Preparation:
- Give meals your full attention and care.
- Being present when preparing meals helps you feel more connected to the food and the process, which improves the whole eating experience.

3. Paying Attention to Cues of Fullness and Hunger:
- Pay attention to your body's signals of hunger and fullness.
- Eat when you're hungry and take short breaks to gauge your level of contentment to avoid mindless, emotionally driven eating.

4. Reducing Distractions:
- Reduce distractions to create a concentrated atmosphere during meals.
- Switch off electronics and avoid multitasking so that you may eat more deliberately and enjoyably.

5. Chewing and Digestion Awareness:
- Chew food well, taking time to appreciate each bite.
   - A better understanding of the chewing process facilitates digestion and strengthens the bond between the body and mind.

6. Practice Gratitude:
- Show appreciation for the food that is on the dish.
   - Acknowledging the labor-intensive process of putting food on the table may help cultivate a grateful and optimistic outlook.

7. Non-Judgmental Observation:
 - Accept the current moment, including any feelings that may occur.
 - Observe thoughts and emotions without passing judgment.
   - This practice fosters a more compassionate relationship with oneself.

Emotional Support through Nutrition:

A well-balanced diet that includes a range of fruits, vegetables, whole grains, lean meats, and healthy fats is recommended for stability.
Foods high in nutrients offer vital vitamins and minerals that promote emotional equilibrium and cognitive function.

Consume foods high in fatty fish, flaxseeds, and walnuts, among other sources of omega-3 fatty acids.
Omega-3 fatty acids have been connected to happier moods and may help with emotional difficulties.

Drink enough water throughout the day. Dehydration can affect mood and cognitive function, therefore it's essential to consume enough fluids.

Reduce intake of excessive stimulants and processed sugars.

Maintaining stable blood sugar levels is essential for maintaining steady energy levels and mental health.

Investigate adaptogenic herbs such as holy basil or ashwagandha.
Adaptogens may support emotional resilience by helping the body adjust to stress.

Permit guilt-free, infrequent pleasures. Intentionally indulging in little pleasures promotes mental and nutritional equilibrium.

To promote social connection, share meals with loved ones. The emotional advantages of mindful eating are increased when food is consumed in a community setting.

Chapter 8

Lifestyle Changes for Long-Term Health

Establishing Sustainable Habits:

Gradual Progression: To boost confidence, start with modest, attainable objectives. Implement changes gradually to give the body and mind time to become used to new routines.

Nutrient-Dense Eating: Adopt a diet that is both balanced and rich in nutrients. Give priority to entire foods in order to supply the necessary nutrients for long-term energy and vigor. These include fruits, vegetables, lean meats, whole grains, and healthy fats.

Mindful Eating Techniques: To improve the awareness and pleasure of meals, engage in mindful eating techniques. Develop a healthy connection with food by learning to appreciate every bite and to recognize signs of hunger and fullness.

Regular Sleep Schedule: Create a regular sleep schedule to ensure that you get enough sleep. Restorative sleep is critical for both mental and physical recuperation and for maintaining general health.

Stress Reduction Methods: Include stress-relieving exercises like yoga, meditation, or deep breathing exercises. Managing stress contributes to emotional well-being and helps prevent the negative impact of chronic stress on health.

Social Connection: Promote deep and meaningful social ties. Participating in a community that offers support enhances emotional health and gives one a feeling of direction.

Constant Learning: Develop an attitude of self-improvement and constant learning. Learning new things and taking on new challenges improve mental health and foster personal development.

Physical Activity and Its Role in Recovery:

- Personalized Exercise Plans:
Seek advice from medical specialists to create customized workout regimens. Take into account variables including fitness levels, medical problems, and recuperation objectives.

- Finding a Balance between Strength and Cardiovascular workouts:
Use a variety of strength and cardiovascular workouts.This combo strengthens muscles, promotes heart health, and improves general fitness.

- Adaptive Exercise:

Investigate exercises that are tailored to certain health concerns. Exercises like yoga, walking, and swimming may be modified to meet different health demands and fitness levels.

- Mind-Body Exercises:

Take part in mind-body activities such as tai chi or yoga. These pursuits enhance mental clarity and physical well-being in addition to lowering stress.

- Frequent Movement Breaks:

Include frequent movement breaks in your everyday schedule. Simple exercises, stretching, and quick walks can assist increase circulation and break up times of inactivity.

- Outdoor Activities:

Take advantage of outdoor activities to get some fresh air and spend time in nature. -

Exercising outside offers extra advantages for mood and mental health.

- Setting Progressive Goals:
Establish attainable yet challenging fitness objectives.
Honor accomplishments, regardless of whether they entail more flexibility, stronger muscles, or greater endurance.

- Include Pleasurable Activities:
Select pleasurable physical pursuits. Finding delight in exercise, whether it be dancing, hiking, or team sports, boosts the probability of sustained commitment.

Smoking Cessation and Limiting Alcohol:

Seek out expert assistance and resources to help you stop smoking. Programs for stopping, counseling, and nicotine replacement therapy can increase your chances of success.

Give smokers access to gradual reduction techniques. A strategy for quitting smoking that works well is gradual decrease together with assistance.

Recognize what sets off a person to smoke or drink too much alcohol. Developing better coping mechanisms requires an understanding of the circumstances or feelings that give rise to these behaviors.

Replace drinking and smoking with better behaviors.Taking up hobbies, exercising, or practicing meditation might offer substitute coping mechanisms for stress or boredom.

Establish reasonable guidelines for alcohol use. Moderation is advised, with one drink for women and two for men per day being the recommended amount.

Include days without alcohol in your weekly schedule. This exercise encourages moderation and gives the body time to heal itself.

Discuss objectives with loved ones, close friends, or support networks. Support and accountability are important factors in the effectiveness of lifestyle modifications, particularly when treating addictive behaviors.

Seek individualized advice from healthcare specialists. Experts can offer customized approaches for reducing alcohol intake and quitting smoking, taking into account each person's requirements and difficulties.

Chapter 9

Eating Throughout the Day: 101 Super & Easy Recipes

Breakfast Recipes:

1. Quinoa Breakfast Bowl

Ingredients:
- 1 cup quinoa
- 2 cups almond milk (or any preferred milk)
- 1 tablespoon honey or maple syrup
- 1 teaspoon vanilla extract
- 1 cup mixed berries (strawberries, blueberries, raspberries)
- 1 banana, sliced
- ¼ cup chopped nuts (almonds, walnuts)
- 1 tablespoon chia seeds
- A pinch of cinnamon
- Greek yogurt (optional, for serving)

Instructions:
- Rinse the quinoa in cold water to get rid of the bitter flavor.

- Put the quinoa and almond milk in a pot. After bringing to a boil, lower the heat to a simmer, cover, and cook the quinoa for 15 to 20 minutes, or until the liquid has been absorbed.

- Turn off the heat and leave it covered for five minutes. Using a fork, fluff the quinoa.

- Combine vanilla extract and honey (or maple syrup) in a small bowl. Pour the liquid over the cooked quinoa and mix it in.

- Spoon quinoa that has been sweetened into serving dishes.

- Add chopped almonds, chia seeds, banana slices, and mixed berries to the top of each bowl.

- Drizzle each dish with a little bit of cinnamon.

- For extra richness, feel free to top the dish with a dollop of Greek yogurt.

2. Avocado Toast with Poached Egg

Ingredients:
- 2 slices whole-grain bread
- 1 ripe avocado
- 2 large eggs
- Salt and pepper to taste
- Red pepper flakes (optional, for added spice)
- Fresh cilantro or parsley, chopped (for garnish)

Instructions:
- Toast the pieces of whole-grain bread until they are as crispy as you like.

Avocado Preparation:
- Halve the ripe avocado, extract the pit, and transfer the flesh to a basin.
- Using a fork, mash the avocado until it becomes creamy.
- Add salt and pepper to taste while seasoning the mashed avocado.

Poach the Eggs:
- Simmer a kettle of water until it is just simmering.
- Crack each egg into a little basin of its own.
- Gently stir the water until it forms a nice vortex, then carefully slip the eggs into the middle.
- If you want a runny yolk, poach the eggs for 3–4 minutes; if you want a firmer yolk, poach for longer.
- The poached eggs may be gently removed from the water by using a slotted spoon.

- To assemble the avocado toast, evenly spread the mashed avocado on top of the toast.

- Top each toast with a poached egg after it has been smeared in avocado.

Season and Garnish:

- If you prefer a little heat, add some red pepper flakes, salt, and pepper to the poached eggs.

- For an extra burst of flavor, sprinkle some freshly chopped parsley or cilantro on top of the avocado toast.

- While the eggs are still warm, serve the avocado toast and poached egg right away.

- Slice into the poached egg so that the yolk may artfully pour over the smooth avocado.

3. Smoothie Bowl

Ingredients:

For the Smoothie:
- 1 frozen banana, sliced
- 1 cup frozen mixed berries (strawberries, blueberries, raspberries)
- ½ cup plain Greek yogurt
- ½ cup almond milk (or any preferred milk)
- 1 tablespoon honey or maple syrup (optional for added sweetness)
- 1 teaspoon chia seeds (optional, for texture)
- ½ teaspoon vanilla extract

For Toppings:
- Sliced fresh fruits (e.g., berries, kiwi, banana)
- Granola
- Chopped nuts (almonds, walnuts)
- Coconut flakes
- Chia seeds

- Drizzle of honey or nut butter (optional)

Instructions:

To make the smoothie, add frozen banana slices, frozen mixed berries, Greek yogurt, almond milk, chia seeds, vanilla extract, and honey (or maple syrup) to a blender. Blend till creamy and smooth. Add extra almond milk if necessary to get the consistency you want.

- Transfer the smoothie into a bowl.

- Top the smoothie with chopped nuts, granola, chia seeds, coconut flakes, and sliced fresh fruit.

- To add sweetness and taste, you can optionally pour almond butter or honey over the toppings.

4. Oatmeal with Nut Butter and Banana

Ingredients:

- ½ cup old-fashioned rolled oats
- 1 cup milk (dairy or plant-based)
- 1 ripe banana, sliced
- 1 tablespoon nut butter (peanut butter, almond butter, or your choice)
- 1 tablespoon honey or maple syrup
- ½ teaspoon ground cinnamon
- A pinch of salt
- Chopped nuts (optional, for garnish)
- Sliced strawberries or berries (optional, for garnish)
- Drizzle of additional honey (optional, for extra sweetness)

Instructions:

- Put the rolled oats and milk in a pot. Once the oats are cooked and the mixture reaches the required thickness, bring it to a mild boil, then lower the heat to a simmer and stir from time to time.

- To gently soften the oats, stir in sliced bananas during the last minute of cooking.

- After the oatmeal has cooked, take it off the stove and mix with some nut butter, honey (or maple syrup), ground cinnamon, and salt.
- Once the nut butter has melted and the ingredients are properly blended, stir vigorously.

- Add a garnish by moving the oatmeal into a bowl.
- Add sliced strawberries (or other berries), chopped almonds, and an optional extra drizzle of honey.

5. Greek Yogurt Parfait

Ingredients:

- 1 cup Greek yogurt
- 1 tablespoon honey or maple syrup
- ½ cup granola
- ½ cup mixed berries (strawberries, blueberries, raspberries)
- 1 tablespoon chia seeds
- ¼ cup chopped nuts (almonds, walnuts)
- Optional: ½ teaspoon vanilla extract
- Optional: Fresh mint leaves for garnish

Instructions:

- To make the Greek yogurt, combine the yogurt with honey (or maple syrup) and vanilla extract, if preferred, in a bowl. This gives your parfait a delicious, creamy basis.

Layer with Granola:
- Spoon a layer of Greek yogurt into a glass or dish to begin creating your parfait.

- Sprinkle some granola over the yogurt.

Add Mixed Berries:
 - Cover the granola with a layer of mixed berries. Maintain a uniform dispersion to achieve a harmonious flavor.

Distribute Chia Seeds:
 - Distribute chia seeds throughout the layer of berries. A wonderful crunch and nutritious boost are added by the chia seeds.

Repeat Layers:
 - Continue layering until the top of the bowl or glass is reached. Since the order is adjustable, you can customize based on your preference.

Top with Nuts:
 - Finish off your parfait with a generous sprinkle of chopped nuts. This adds a delightful texture and nutty flavor.

Garnish (Optional):

- Optionally, garnish with fresh mint leaves for a burst of freshness.

6. Veggie Omelette for Breast Cancer Diet

Ingredients:

- 2 large eggs
- ¼ cup diced bell peppers (mix of colors)
- ¼ cup diced tomatoes
- ¼ cup chopped spinach
- ¼ cup diced red onions
- ¼ cup sliced mushrooms
- 1 tablespoon olive oil
- Salt and pepper to taste
- Fresh herbs (such as parsley or chives) for garnish
- Optional: Feta cheese or goat cheese (for added flavor)

Instructions:

- Chop bell peppers, tomatoes, red onions, and slice mushrooms as you prepare the vegetables.
- Chop the spinach and reserve.

Sauté Vegetables:
- Heat olive oil in a nonstick pan over medium heat.
- Sauté the red onions until they become transparent.
- Add the spinach, tomatoes, bell peppers, and mushrooms. Sauté the veggies till they get soft.

Whisk Eggs:
- Beat the eggs together thoroughly in a bowl.
- Add pepper and salt for seasoning.

Prepare the Omelet:
- Spoon the scrambled eggs into the pan of sautéed veggies.

- After letting the edges solidify, carefully raise them with a spatula to allow the raw egg to seep below.

Add Optional Cheese:
- You can choose to top half of the omelet with crumbled goat or feta cheese.

Fold and Serve:
- Gently fold the omelet in half once the eggs are largely set but still little runny on top.
- Cook for a minute more, or until the eggs are set and the cheese has melted.

Arrange and Savor:
- Transfer the Vegetable Omelet onto a dish.
- If wanted, garnish with more pepper and fresh herbs.

7. Chia Seed Pudding

Ingredients:

- ¼ cup chia seeds
- 1 cup almond milk (or any preferred milk)
- 1 tablespoon honey or maple syrup
- ½ teaspoon vanilla extract
- Fresh berries (strawberries, blueberries, raspberries) for topping
- Sliced almonds or chopped nuts for topping
- Optional: Greek yogurt for layering
- Optional: A pinch of cinnamon for flavor

Instructions:

Blend Almond Milk and Chia Seeds:
   - Place chia seeds and almond milk in a bowl. A good stir will prevent clumping.

Add Sweeteners and Flavor:
   - Incorporate vanilla essence and honey (or maple syrup) into the chia seed mixture.

- For added taste, feel free to add a pinch of cinnamon.

Stir and Chill:
- Give the mixture a good stir, then cover the dish or portion it out into separate jars.
- To enable the chia seeds to absorb the liquid and take on the consistency of pudding, refrigerate for at least two to three hours, or overnight.

Optional Greek Yogurt Layer:
- To add even more richness, fill serving glasses with chia pudding and Greek yogurt.

Cover with Fresh Berries and Nuts:
- After the chia pudding has firmed, cover it with a layer of fresh berries and a scattering of chopped nuts or sliced almonds.

Present and Savor:
- Present the Chia Seed Pudding in a cooled state.

- Before consuming, combine the layers to savor the exquisite blend of flavors and textures.

8. Pancakes with Maple Syrup

Ingredients:

- 1 cup all-purpose flour
- 2 tablespoons sugar
- 1 teaspoon baking powder
- ½ teaspoon baking soda
- ¼ teaspoon salt
- ¾ cup buttermilk
- 1 large egg
- 2 tablespoons unsalted butter, melted
- 1 teaspoon vanilla extract
- Cooking spray or additional butter for greasing the pan
- Maple syrup for serving

Instructions:

- To prepare the dry ingredients, mix together the flour, sugar, baking soda, baking powder, and salt in a large basin.

Combine Wet Ingredients:
- Beat buttermilk, egg, melted butter, and vanilla extract in another dish.

Incorporate Wet and Dry Ingredients: - Transfer the wet components into the dry components. Mix until well blended; a few lumps are good. Avoid over-mixing.

Heat the Pan:
- Turn on a nonstick pan or griddle to medium heat. Apply butter or frying spray to lightly grease.

Cook the Pancakes:
- For each pancake, pour ¼ cup of batter onto the griddle.

- Cook until surface bubbles appear, then turn and continue cooking until golden brown on the other side.

- To serve warm, stack the pancakes onto a dish and maintain their warmth.
   - Drizzle plenty of maple syrup over the pancakes before serving.

Optional Toppings:
   - Garnish your pancakes with extras like chopped bananas, fresh berries, or a scoop of Greek yogurt.

9. Fruit and Nut Smoothie

Ingredients:

- 1 banana, peeled and sliced
- ½ cup frozen mixed berries (strawberries, blueberries, raspberries)
- ¼ cup Greek yogurt
- 1 tablespoon almond butter

- 1 tablespoon chia seeds
- 1 tablespoon honey or maple syrup
- 1 cup almond milk (or any preferred milk)
- ¼ cup rolled oats
- Ice cubes (optional, for a colder smoothie)

Instructions:

- Slice the banana and measure the rolled oats, almond milk, Greek yogurt, honey (or maple syrup), chia seeds, almond butter, and frozen mixed berries.

Combine in Blender:
- Place the frozen mixed berries, Greek yogurt, almond butter, chia seeds, banana slices, rolled oats, honey (or maple syrup), and almond milk in a blender.

Blend till Smooth:
- Process the mixture in a blender until it becomes creamy and smooth. To make the smoothie cooler, feel free to add ice cubes.

Adjust Thickness:
- If the smoothie is too thick, mix in a small amount of extra almond milk at a time until the right thickness is achieved.

- Pour the fruit and nut smoothie into a glass and serve immediately.

Optional Garnish:
- For an added touch, scatter some chia seeds or a few whole berries on top.

Customize:
- You may add extra nutrients to the smoothie by adding a handful of spinach or your preferred nuts or seeds.

10. Whole Grain Waffles

Ingredients:

- 1 cup whole wheat flour
- ½ cup all-purpose flour

- 2 tablespoons sugar
- 1 tablespoon baking powder
- ½ teaspoon salt
- 1½ cups milk (dairy or plant-based)
- ⅓ cup vegetable oil or melted coconut oil
- 2 large eggs
- 1 teaspoon vanilla extract
- Cooking spray or additional oil for greasing the waffle iron
- Toppings: Fresh berries, sliced bananas, maple syrup, or Greek yogurt (optional)

Instructions:

Waffle Iron Prep:
  - Follow the manufacturer's directions to preheat your waffle iron.

Combine Dry Ingredients:
  - In a sizable bowl, mix together sugar, baking powder, salt, whole wheat flour, and all-purpose flour.

Mix Wet Ingredients:
- Beat together milk, eggs, vegetable oil, and vanilla essence in a separate basin.

Incorporate Wet and Dry Ingredients:
- Transfer the wet components into the dry components. Mix until well blended; a few lumps are OK. Avoid over-mixing.

Grease the Waffle Iron:
- Apply a thin layer of cooking spray or oil to the waffle iron.

Prepare the waffles by:
- Covering the waffle grid with enough batter on the hot waffle iron. Once the waffles are golden brown, close the waffle iron and cook them as directed by the manufacturer.

- Warm waffles should be served by carefully removing them from the iron and repeating the process with the remaining batter.

- Top the heated Whole Grain Waffles with your preferred garnishes.

Lunch Recipes:

1. Quinoa Salad with Chickpeas

Ingredients:

For the Salad:
- 1 cup quinoa, rinsed
- 2 cups water
- 1 can (15 oz) chickpeas, drained and rinsed
- 1 cucumber, diced
- 1 bell pepper (any color), diced
- 1 cup cherry tomatoes, halved
- ¼ cup red onion, finely chopped
- ¼ cup feta cheese, crumbled (optional)
- ¼ cup fresh parsley, chopped

For the Dressing:
- ¼ cup extra-virgin olive oil
- 2 tablespoons red wine vinegar
- 1 teaspoon Dijon mustard
- 1 clove garlic, minced
- Salt and pepper to taste

Instructions:

Cook Quinoa:
   - Add water to the quinoa in a saucepan. After bringing to a boil, lower heat to a simmer, cover, and cook the quinoa for 15 to 20 minutes, or until it is tender and the water has been absorbed. Take it off the heat and leave it covered for five minutes. Using a fork, fluff the quinoa and set aside to chill.

Assemble the vegetables and chickpeas:
   - The cooked quinoa, chickpeas, chopped bell pepper, diced cucumber, cherry tomatoes, red onion, and crumbled feta cheese (if using) should all be combined in a big bowl.

Prepare the Dressing:
 - Combine the olive oil, red wine vinegar, Dijon mustard, minced garlic, salt, and pepper in a small bowl.

Mix and Toss:
 - Drizzle the quinoa and veggie combination with the dressing.
 - Toss the ingredients in the dressing until well covered.

Chill and Marinate:
- To let the flavors infuse, place the Quinoa Salad in the refrigerator for a minimum of half an hour.

Garnish and Serve:
 - Sprinkle the salad with freshly cut parsley right before serving.

2. Grilled Chicken Caesar Wrap

Ingredients:

For the Grilled Chicken:
- 2 boneless, skinless chicken breasts
- 1 tablespoon olive oil
- 1 teaspoon garlic powder
- 1 teaspoon dried oregano
- Salt and pepper to taste

For the Caesar Dressing:
- ½ cup mayonnaise
- ¼ cup grated Parmesan cheese
- 1 tablespoon Dijon mustard
- 1 tablespoon lemon juice
- 1 clove garlic, minced
- Salt and pepper to taste

For the Wrap:
- 4 whole wheat or spinach tortillas
- Romaine lettuce leaves, washed and dried
- 1 cup cherry tomatoes, halved
- ¼ cup sliced black olives (optional)

- ¼ cup grated Parmesan cheese
- Additional Caesar dressing for drizzling

Instructions:

Grill the Chicken:
 - Turn up the heat to medium-high on the grill or grill pan.
   - Garlic powder, dried oregano, olive oil, salt, and pepper should be applied to the chicken breasts.
   - Cook the chicken for 6 to 8 minutes on each side, or until it's well done. Before slicing, let it rest for a few minutes.

   - Prepare the Caesar Dressing by whisking together the mayonnaise, lemon juice, chopped garlic, Dijon mustard, grated Parmesan cheese, salt, and pepper in a bowl. Taste and adjust the seasoning.

Put the Wrap Together:
- Arrange the tortillas on a level surface.

- Dot each tortilla with a heaping scoop of Caesar dressing.

Add the Chicken and Toppings:
 - Center each tortilla with a piece of grilled chicken.
 - Top with grated Parmesan cheese, cherry tomatoes, chopped black olives (if using), and Romaine lettuce leaves.

Drizzle with Dressing:
 - Spoon extra Caesar dressing on top of the ingredients.

Fold and Serve:
 - Tightly roll the tortilla to form a wrap by folding the edges over the filling.
 - If necessary, secure them with toothpicks.

3. Stuffed Bell Peppers with Quinoa

Ingredients:

- 4 large bell peppers, halved and seeds removed
- 1 cup quinoa, rinsed
- 2 cups vegetable broth or water
- 1 tablespoon olive oil
- 1 onion, finely chopped
- 2 cloves garlic, minced
- 1 zucchini, diced
- 1 cup cherry tomatoes, halved
- 1 can (15 oz) black beans, drained and rinsed
- 1 teaspoon ground cumin
- 1 teaspoon smoked paprika
- Salt and pepper to taste
- 1 cup shredded cheese (cheddar, Monterey Jack, or your choice)
- Fresh cilantro or parsley for garnish

Instructions:

Oven Prep:
- Set the oven's temperature to 375°F, or 190°C.

- Prepare the bell peppers by cutting them in half lengthwise and removing the membranes and seeds.
- Put them inside a dish for baking.

Prepare the Quinoa:
- Put the Quinoa and the veggie broth (or water) in a pot. After bringing to a boil, lower heat, cover, and simmer the quinoa for 15 to 20 minutes, or until it is tender and the liquid has been absorbed. Using a fork, fluff.

Sauté Vegetables:
- Heat olive oil in a big pan over medium heat. Add the chopped onion and garlic, and cook them until they become soft. Add the black beans, cherry tomatoes, and sliced

zucchini. Sauté the veggies for a further three to five minutes, or until they are soft.

Season and Mix:
- Add salt, pepper, smoked paprika, and ground cumin.
- Mix the cooked quinoa with the sautéed veggies.

Stuff Bell Peppers:
- Gently push down on each half of the bell pepper after adding a small amount of the quinoa and veggie mixture.
- Top each filled pepper with grated cheese.

Bake:
- Bake the peppers for 25 to 30 minutes, or until they are soft, while covering the baking dish with foil.

Garnish and Serve:
- Take out of the oven and sprinkle with chopped parsley or cilantro.

- Warm quinoa should be served with stuffed bell peppers.

4. Mediterranean Chickpea Salad

Ingredients:

- 2 cans (15 oz each) chickpeas, drained and rinsed
- 1 cup cherry tomatoes, halved
- 1 cucumber, diced
- ½ red onion, finely chopped
- ½ cup Kalamata olives, sliced
- ½ cup crumbled feta cheese
- ¼ cup fresh parsley, chopped

For the Dressing:
- ¼ cup extra-virgin olive oil
- 2 tablespoons red wine vinegar
- 1 teaspoon dried oregano
- 1 clove garlic, minced
- Salt and pepper to taste

Instructions:

Cook the Chickpeas:
 - Put the rinsed and drained chickpeas in a big bowl.

Add the Vegetables:
 - Fill the bowl with cherry tomatoes, sliced Kalamata olives, diced cucumber, minced red onion, and crumbled feta cheese.

Prepare the Dressing:
 - Combine the extra virgin olive oil, red wine vinegar, minced garlic, dried oregano, salt, and pepper in a small dish.

Combine and Toss:
 - Drizzle the chickpea and veggie mixture with the dressing.
 - Gently toss the ingredients until the dressing coats everything.

- To enable the flavors to mingle, place the Mediterranean Chickpea Salad in the refrigerator for at least half an hour.

Garnish and Serve:
 - Just before serving, top the salad with freshly cut parsley.

5. Veggie and Hummus Wrap

Ingredients:

- 4 whole wheat or spinach tortillas
- 1 cup hummus (store-bought or homemade)
- 1 cup baby spinach leaves
- 1 cucumber, julienned
- 1 bell pepper (any color), thinly sliced
- 1 carrot, julienned or shredded
- ½ red onion, thinly sliced
- 1 avocado, sliced
- Sprouts or microgreens for garnish (optional)

- Salt and pepper to taste

Instructions:

- To prepare the ingredients, spread the tortillas out on a level surface.

Spread Hummus:
- Evenly cover each tortilla with a good portion of hummus.

Add the Vegetables and Spinach:
- Sprinkle some baby spinach leaves over the hummus.
- Arrange pieces of avocado, bell pepper, carrot, cucumber, and red onion on top of the spinach.

Add a dash of salt and pepper to taste:
- Add a dash of salt and pepper to the veggies.

Sprouts as an Optional Garnish:
   - For a crisp and fresh garnish, feel free to add microgreens or sprouts.

Wrap and Serve:
  - Gently tuck the tortilla's edges in and roll it firmly from the bottom to form a wrap.

Cut and Savor:
   - Cut the Hummus and Vegetables Wrap in a diagonal fashion for easy handling.

6. Salmon and Quinoa Bowl

Ingredients:

For the Salmon:
- 4 salmon filets
- 2 tablespoons olive oil
- 1 teaspoon smoked paprika
- 1 teaspoon garlic powder
- Salt and pepper to taste
- Lemon wedges for serving

For the Quinoa:
- 1 cup quinoa, rinsed
- 2 cups vegetable broth or water
- 1 tablespoon lemon juice
- Salt to taste

For the Bowl:
- 2 cups baby spinach leaves
- 1 cucumber, sliced
- 1 avocado, sliced
- 1 cup cherry tomatoes, halved
- ¼ cup red onion, finely chopped
- ¼ cup feta cheese, crumbled
- Fresh parsley for garnish

For the Dressing:
- 3 tablespoons extra-virgin olive oil
- 1 tablespoon balsamic vinegar
- 1 teaspoon Dijon mustard
- Salt and pepper to taste

Instructions:

- In order to prepare the salmon, preheat the oven to 400°F, or 200°C.
- Salmon filets should be rubbed with olive oil, salt, pepper, garlic powder, and smoky paprika.
- Arrange the filets onto a parchment paper-lined baking sheet.
- Bake the salmon for 12 to 15 minutes, or until it is cooked through and flakes readily when tested with a fork.

Prepare Quinoa:
- Put quinoa and vegetable broth (or water) in a pot. After bringing to a boil, lower heat, cover, and simmer the quinoa for 15 to 20 minutes, or until it is tender and the liquid has been absorbed.
- Using a fork, fluff the quinoa and season with salt and lemon juice.

Prepare the Vegetables:
- Combine the avocado, cherry tomatoes, red onion, cucumber slices, baby spinach, and crumbled feta cheese in a bowl.

- To make the dressing, combine the extra virgin olive oil, balsamic vinegar, Dijon mustard, salt, and pepper in a small bowl.

Put the Bowl Together:
- Spoon the cooked quinoa into each of the serving dishes.
Place the veggie mixture and a cooked salmon filet on top.

Dressing Drizzle:
- Cover the bowl with a balsamic Dijon dressing drizzle.

Garnish and Serve:
- Add some fresh parsley as a garnish.
- Present the Quinoa and Salmon Bowl accompanied by slices of lemon.

7. Caprese Pasta Salad

Ingredients:

- 8 oz (about 2 cups) cherry tomatoes, halved
- 1 cup fresh mozzarella balls (bocconcini), halved
- ¼ cup fresh basil leaves, torn
- ¼ cup extra-virgin olive oil
- 2 tablespoons balsamic vinegar
- 2 cloves garlic, minced
- Salt and pepper to taste
- 8 oz (about 2 cups) pasta (penne, fusilli, or your choice)
- Balsamic glaze for drizzling (optional)

Instructions:

- To prepare pasta, follow the directions on the package to cook it until it reaches al dente.

- To cool down, drain and rinse with cold water.

Mix Tomatoes, Mozzarella, and Basil:
- Put the halved cherry tomatoes, fresh mozzarella balls, and shredded basil leaves in a big bowl.

Prepare the Dressing:
- Combine extra virgin olive oil, balsamic vinegar, minced garlic, salt, and pepper in a small bowl.

Combine Pasta and Vegetables:
- Include tomatoes, mozzarella, and basil in a dish with the chilled pasta.

Drizzle with Dressing:
- Drizzle the pasta and veggies with the dressing.
- Mix everything until well combined.

- To let the flavors infuse, place the Caprese Pasta Salad in the refrigerator for a minimum of half an hour.

Drizzle with Balsamic Glaze (Optional):
 - To provide an extra flavor boost, drizzle with balsamic glaze right before serving.

8. Vegetarian Sushi Rolls

Ingredients:

For the Sushi Rice:
- 1 cup sushi rice
- 1¼ cups water
- ¼ cup rice vinegar
- 2 tablespoons sugar
- 1 teaspoon salt

For the Vegetarian Filling:
- 1 avocado, sliced
- 1 cucumber, julienned
- 1 carrot, julienned

- 1 bell pepper (any color), thinly sliced
- 10 sheets nori (seaweed)

For Dipping Sauce:
- Soy sauce
- Wasabi (optional)
- Pickled ginger (optional)

Instructions:

- Sushi rice should be prepared by rinsing it under cold water until the water runs clear.

- In a saucepan or rice cooker, combine rice and water. Follow the directions on the package to cook.

- Rice vinegar, sugar, and salt should be heated in a small saucepan over low heat until the sugar dissolves. Give it time to cool.

- After the rice is cooked, pour it into a big bowl and mix in the seasoned rice vinegar with a gentle stir. Let the rice cool until it reaches room temperature.

Prepare the vegetables:
- Finely slice the bell pepper, julienne the cucumber, julienne the avocado, and so on.

Assemble Sushi Rolls:
- Lay down a bamboo sushi rolling mat on a level surface. - Place a nori sheet, shiny side down, on the mat.
- Using wet hands, distribute around one cup of sushi rice evenly over the nori, leaving a small border at the top.
- In the center of the rice, arrange a few slices of bell pepper, cucumber, avocado, and carrot.

Roll the Sushi:
- Using the bamboo mat, gently press the sushi away from you as you raise and roll it securely, starting from the bottom.
- To seal the roll, wet the upper edge of the nori with water.

Slice the Roll:

- Cut the sushi roll into bite-sized pieces using a sharp, damp knife.

9. Turkey and Quinoa Stuffed Peppers

Ingredients:

- 4 large bell peppers, halved and seeds removed
- 1 cup quinoa, rinsed
- 2 cups vegetable broth or water
- 1 tablespoon olive oil
- 1 onion, finely chopped
- 2 cloves garlic, minced
- 1 pound ground turkey
- 1 can (15 oz) black beans, drained and rinsed
- 1 cup corn kernels (fresh or frozen)
- 1 teaspoon ground cumin
- 1 teaspoon chili powder
- Salt and pepper to taste
- 1 cup shredded cheese (cheddar or Mexican blend)

- Fresh cilantro for garnish

Instructions:

Oven Prep:
 - Set the oven's temperature to 375°F, or 190°C.

 - Prepare the bell peppers by cutting them in half lengthwise and removing the membranes and seeds. Put them inside a dish for baking.

Prepare the Quinoa:
 - Put the Quinoa and the veggie broth (or water) in a pot. After bringing to a boil, lower heat, cover, and simmer the quinoa for 15 to 20 minutes, or until it is tender and the liquid has been absorbed.
 - Using a fork, fluff the quinoa and set it aside.

Sauté the onion and garlic:
- Heat the olive oil in a big pan over medium heat. Add the chopped onion and garlic, and cook until they become soft.

Cook the Turkey:
- Fill the skillet with the ground turkey and cook it until browned, breaking it up with a spoon as it cooks.

- Add the corn and black beans, stirring to combine. Also add the chili powder, ground cumin, salt, and pepper. Cook for a further three to five minutes, or until well heated.

Stir Quinoa and Turkey Mixture Together:
- Stir the cooked quinoa into the turkey mixture.

Stuffed Peppers:
- Fill each bell pepper half half half to the brim with the turkey and quinoa mixture.

Add Cheese on Top:
 - Drizzle the filled peppers with shredded cheese.

Bake:
 - Bake the peppers for 25 to 30 minutes, or until they are soft, while covering the baking dish with foil.

Garnish and Serve:
- Take the turkey and quinoa stuffed peppers out of the oven, top with some fresh cilantro, and serve them hot.

10. Veggie Stir-Fry with Tofu:

Ingredients:
- 1 block firm tofu, pressed and cubed
- 2 cups broccoli florets
- 1 bell pepper, thinly sliced
- 1 carrot, julienned
- 1 cup snap peas, ends trimmed
- 3 tablespoons soy sauce

- 1 tablespoon sesame oil
- 2 tablespoons vegetable oil
- 2 cloves garlic, minced
- 1 tablespoon ginger, grated
- 1 tablespoon rice vinegar
- 1 tablespoon cornstarch (optional, for extra thickness)
- Sesame seeds and green onions for garnish
- Cooked brown rice or quinoa for serving

Method:

- Tofu preparation involves pressing it to squeeze out extra water.
- Chop the tofu into small pieces.

Stir-Fry Tofu:
- In a large pan, heat the vegetable oil over medium-high heat.
When the tofu cubes get golden brown on both sides, add them.
- Take out the tofu and place it aside.

Sauté Aromatics:
 - If necessary, add a little extra oil to the same pan.
 - Fry grated ginger and chopped garlic until aromatic.

Cook the Vegetables:
- Add the snap peas, carrot, bell pepper, and broccoli to the pan.
 - Stir-fry the veggies until they become crisp-tender.

Mix Tofu and veggies:
 - Add the cooked tofu and veggies back to the pan.

Prepare Sauce:
 - Combine rice vinegar, sesame oil, and soy sauce in a bowl.
 - Add cornstarch to the sauce after mixing it with a little amount of water if you'd like it thicker.

Drizzle Sauce Over Stir-Fry:
- Drizzle the sauce over the veggies and tofu.
- Combine all the ingredients, making sure the tofu and veggies are equally coated in sauce.

- To serve, cook for a further two to three minutes, or until everything is well cooked.
- Add chopped green onions and sesame seeds as garnish.

Top with Quinoa or Rice:
- Serve the cooked quinoa or brown rice with the veggie stir-fry with tofu on top.

Dinner Recipes:

1. Grilled Lemon Herb Chicken

Ingredients:

- 4 boneless, skinless chicken breasts
- Zest and juice of 2 lemons
- 3 tablespoons olive oil
- 2 cloves garlic, minced
- 1 teaspoon dried oregano
- 1 teaspoon dried thyme
- 1 teaspoon dried rosemary
- Salt and pepper to taste
- Lemon slices for garnish (optional)
- Fresh herbs (parsley, thyme, or rosemary) for garnish

Instructions:

- To marinade the chicken, combine the lemon zest, lemon juice, olive oil, minced garlic, dried thyme, dried rosemary, dried oregano, and salt and pepper in a dish.

- Pour the marinade over the chicken breasts and place them in a shallow dish or zip-top bag. Make sure the chicken has a good coating.

- For optimal taste, marinate it for up to 4 hours, but at least 30 minutes should be spent in the fridge.

Preheat the Grill:
- Turn the heat up to medium-high.

Grill the Chicken:
- Take the chicken out of the marinade and let any extra to fall off.

- After preheating the grill, place the chicken on it and cook it for 6 to 8 minutes on each side, or until it is cooked through and the internal temperature reaches 165°F (74°C).

Baste with Marinade:
- To keep the chicken juicy and tasty while it's cooking, baste it with the leftover marinade.

Rest and Garnish:

 - After the chicken has finished cooking, move it to a platter and give it a few minutes to rest. Add fresh herbs and slices of lemon as garnish.

Serve:

 - Arrange your preferred side dishes to go with the Grilled Lemon Herb Chicken.

2. Vegetarian Chickpea Curry

Ingredients:

- 2 cans (15 oz each) chickpeas, drained and rinsed
- 2 tablespoons vegetable oil
- 1 large onion, finely chopped
- 3 cloves garlic, minced
- 1 tablespoon fresh ginger, grated
- 1 tablespoon curry powder
- 1 teaspoon ground cumin

- 1 teaspoon ground coriander
- ½ teaspoon turmeric powder
- ¼ teaspoon cayenne pepper (adjust to taste)
- 1 can (14 oz) diced tomatoes
- 1 can (13.5 oz) coconut milk
- Salt and pepper to taste
- Fresh cilantro for garnish
- Cooked rice or naan for serving

Instructions:

Sauté Aromatics:
 - Heat vegetable oil in a big pan or skillet over medium heat. When the onion is soft, add it to the diced and sauté it.

Add Garlic and Ginger:
 - Fill the pan with grated ginger and chopped garlic. Sauté until aromatic, one or two more minutes.

Spice Blend:

- Blend in cayenne pepper, turmeric powder, powdered coriander, cumin, and curry powder. To bring out the flavors, cook the spices for one to two minutes.

Mix Tomatoes and Chickpeas:

- Pour the rinsed and drained chickpeas into the pan and coat them with the spice mixture.
- Add the chopped tomatoes together with their juice. Mix well to blend.

Simmer with Coconut Milk:

- To make a creamy curry base, pour in the coconut milk and stir.
- To enable the flavors to mingle, bring the mixture to a simmer and cook for 15 to 20 minutes.

Season and Garnish:

- Add salt and pepper to taste when preparing the chickpea curry.

Add some fresh cilantro as a garnish.

Serve:

- You may serve the vegetarian chickpea curry with naan bread or over-boiled rice.

3. Baked Zucchini Boats

Ingredients:

- 4 medium-sized zucchini
- 1 tablespoon olive oil
- ½ cup onion, finely chopped
- 2 cloves garlic, minced
- ½ cup red bell pepper, finely chopped
- ½ cup cherry tomatoes, diced
- 1 cup cooked quinoa or rice
- ½ cup black beans, drained and rinsed
- 1 teaspoon dried oregano
- 1 teaspoon dried basil
- Salt and pepper to taste
- 1 cup shredded mozzarella cheese
- Fresh parsley for garnish

Instructions:

Oven Prep:
 - Set the oven's temperature to 375°F, or 190°C.

Prepare the Zucchini:
 - Halve each one lengthwise. Using a spoon, remove the cores, leaving about 1/2 inch of flesh surrounding the edges. Save the flesh from the zucchini for later.

Sauté Vegetables:
 - Heat olive oil in a pan over medium heat. Add the chopped onion and cook it until it becomes tender. Add the chopped zucchini flesh, red bell pepper, and minced garlic. Cook the veggies for a further three to five minutes, or until they are soft.

Combine Filling:
 - Add cooked quinoa or rice, black beans, dried oregano, dried basil, salt, and pepper

to a dish along with the sautéed veggies. Blend well.

- To fill the zucchini boats, place them in a baking dish.
- Evenly spoon filling mixture into every zucchini boat.

Add Cheese on Top:
- Drizzle the packed zucchini boats with shredded mozzarella cheese.

Bake:
- Bake for 20 to 25 minutes in a preheated oven, or until the cheese is golden and melted and the zucchini is soft.

Garnish and Serve:
- Take out of the oven and sprinkle with parsley that has just been picked.

4. Salmon and Asparagus Foil Packets

Ingredients:

- 4 salmon filets
- 1 bunch asparagus, trimmed
- 1 lemon, thinly sliced
- 4 cloves garlic, minced
- 2 tablespoons fresh dill, chopped
- 2 tablespoons olive oil
- Salt and pepper to taste
- Lemon wedges for serving

Instructions:

Oven Prep:
  - Set the oven's temperature to 400°F, or 200°C.

  - Assemble the foil packets by cutting four sizable pieces of foil.
  - Center each foil piece with a salmon filet.

Season Salmon:
 - Sprinkle salt, pepper, chopped dill, and minced garlic over each filet of salmon.

Add Asparagus and Lemon:
 - Surround each salmon filet with a few handfuls of cut asparagus.
 - Top each salmon filet with a few slices of lemon.

Drizzle with Olive Oil:
 - Drizzle each asparagus spear and salmon filet with a little olive oil.

 - To seal the foil packets containing the salmon and asparagus, fold the foil's edges over the ingredients. Make sure the seal is tight to preserve the taste.

Bake:
 - Put the foil packets on a baking sheet and bake for 15 to 20 minutes, or until the salmon flakes easily, in a preheated oven.

- To serve, carefully unwrap the foil packages while being mindful of the steaming hot food.

- Present the foil packets of salmon and asparagus along with extra lemon wedges.

5. Quinoa Stuffed Bell Peppers

Ingredients:

- 4 large bell peppers, halved and seeds removed
- 1 cup quinoa, rinsed
- 2 cups vegetable broth or water
- 1 tablespoon olive oil
- 1 onion, finely chopped
- 2 cloves garlic, minced
- 1 zucchini, diced
- 1 carrot, grated
- 1 can (14 oz) diced tomatoes, drained
- 1 can (15 oz) black beans, drained and rinsed
- 1 teaspoon ground cumin

- 1 teaspoon chili powder
- Salt and pepper to taste
- 1 cup shredded cheese (cheddar or Mexican blend)
- Fresh cilantro for garnish

Instructions:

Oven Prep:
 - Set the oven's temperature to 375°F, or 190°C.

 - Get the bell peppers ready by cutting each one in half lengthwise. Take out the membranes and seeds.

Prepare the Quinoa:
 - Put the Quinoa and the veggie broth (or water) in a pot. After bringing to a boil, lower heat, cover, and simmer the quinoa for 15 to 20 minutes, or until it is tender and the liquid has been absorbed.

Sauté Vegetables:
 - Heat olive oil in a big pan over medium heat. Add the chopped onion and cook it until it becomes tender. Add the grated carrot, chopped zucchini, and minced garlic. Sauté the veggies for a further three to five minutes, or until they are soft.

Mix Filling:
 - Place cooked quinoa, diced tomatoes, sautéed veggies, ground cumin, chili powder, salt, and pepper in a big bowl. Blend well.

Stuff Bell Peppers:
- Gently push the quinoa and veggie mixture into each side of the bell pepper.

Add Cheese on Top:
 - Drizzle the packed bell peppers with shredded cheese.

Bake:

- In a baking dish, arrange the filled bell peppers. Bake for 25 to 30 minutes in a preheated oven, or until the cheese is bubbling and melted and the peppers are soft.

Garnish and Serve:

- Take out of the oven and top with a handful of fresh cilantro.

- Warm Quinoa Stuffed Bell Peppers should be served.

6. Teriyaki Tofu Stir-Fry

Ingredients:

For the Teriyaki Sauce:
- ¼ cup soy sauce
- 2 tablespoons mirin
- 2 tablespoons rice vinegar
- 1 tablespoon brown sugar
- 1 teaspoon sesame oil

- 1 teaspoon grated ginger
- 2 cloves garlic, minced
- 1 tablespoon cornstarch (optional, for thickening)

For the Stir-Fry:
- 1 block extra-firm tofu, pressed and cubed
- 2 tablespoons vegetable oil
- 1 broccoli crown, cut into florets
- 1 bell pepper, thinly sliced
- 1 carrot, julienned
- 1 cup snow peas, trimmed
- 4 green onions, sliced
- Sesame seeds for garnish (optional)
- Cooked rice for serving

Instructions:

- In a bowl, combine soy sauce, mirin, rice vinegar, brown sugar, sesame oil, grated ginger, and chopped garlic to make the Teriyaki Sauce. Stir in cornstarch for a richer sauce if desired.

Press and Cube Tofu:
  - Press the tofu to get rid of extra moisture. Cube it.

  - Tofu chunks should be tossed in a few teaspoons of teriyaki sauce to marinate. Give it at least fifteen minutes to marinate.

Stir-Fry Tofu:
  - Heat vegetable oil in a large pan or wok over medium-high heat.
  - After adding, stir-fry the marinated tofu until it turns golden brown on both sides. Take out the tofu and place it aside.

Cook the Vegetables:
  - If necessary, add a little extra oil to the same pan. Add the bell pepper, broccoli, julienned carrot, and snow peas and stir-fry until they become crisp-tender.

Mix Tofu and veggies:
  - Return the cooked tofu and veggies to the pan.

Pour Teriyaki Sauce:
- Drizzle the tofu and veggies with the leftover teriyaki sauce. Toss everything in the delicious sauce, giving it a good stir.

- Toss everything together and add the chopped green onions to finish and garnish.
- Garnish the stir-fry with sesame seeds, if preferred.

Serve:
- For a tasty and filling supper, serve the Teriyaki Tofu Stir-Fry over cooked rice.

7. Eggplant Parmesan

Ingredients:

For the Marinara Sauce:
- 2 cans (14 oz each) crushed tomatoes
- 2 cloves garlic, minced
- 1 teaspoon dried oregano
- 1 teaspoon dried basil

- ½ teaspoon salt
- ¼ teaspoon black pepper
- 1 tablespoon olive oil

For the Eggplant:
- 2 large eggplants, sliced into ½ -inch rounds
- Salt for sweating eggplant
- 1 cup all-purpose flour
- 3 large eggs, beaten
- 2 cups breadcrumbs
- 1 cup grated Parmesan cheese
- Vegetable oil for frying

For Assembly:
- 2 cups shredded mozzarella cheese
- ½ cup grated Parmesan cheese
- Fresh basil leaves for garnish

Instructions:

- To make the marinara sauce, place a pot over medium heat and add the olive oil. When aromatic, add the minced garlic and sauté it. Add salt, pepper, dried basil, dry oregano, and smashed tomatoes. Simmer for twenty to thirty minutes, stirring now and again.

Prepare the eggplants:
- Cut them into rounds and season each slice with salt. After letting them perspire for around half an hour, pat them dry.

Breading Station:
- Assemble three shallow dishes: one containing flour, another containing beaten eggs, and a third containing a mixture of breadcrumbs and grated Parmesan cheese.

Bread Eggplant:
- Coat each slice of eggplant with a combination of bread crumbs and Parmesan cheese after dredging it in flour and dipping it into beaten eggs.

- To fry the eggplant, heat up the vegetable oil in a big pan over medium-high heat.

Once both sides are golden brown, fry the breaded eggplant slices. Lay them out on paper towels to soak up extra oil.

Assemble the Layers:
- Turn the oven on to 375°F, or 190°C.
- Cover the bottom of a baking dish with marinara sauce. Add a few pieces of fried eggplant on top. Add grated Parmesan and shredded mozzarella as garnish.
- Continue layering, and then top everything up with a thick covering of cheese.

Bake:
- Bake for 25 to 30 minutes, or until the cheese is bubbling and melted, in a preheated oven.

Garnish and Serve:
- Take it out of the oven and let it rest for a few minutes. Add some fresh basil leaves as garnish.

8. Lentil and Vegetable Stew

Ingredients:

- 1 cup dry green or brown lentils, rinsed and drained
- 2 tablespoons olive oil
- 1 onion, finely chopped
- 2 carrots, diced
- 2 celery stalks, diced
- 3 cloves garlic, minced
- 1 teaspoon ground cumin
- 1 teaspoon ground coriander
- ½ teaspoon smoked paprika
- ½ teaspoon dried thyme
- 1 can (14 oz) diced tomatoes
- 4 cups vegetable broth
- 1 bay leaf
- Salt and pepper to taste
- 2 cups chopped kale or spinach
- Fresh parsley for garnish

Instructions:

- To prepare the lentils, rinse them in cold water and then drain them.

Sauté Vegetables:
- Place a large saucepan over medium heat with olive oil. Add diced celery, diced carrots, and chopped onion. Sauté the veggies till they get tender.

Add Aromatics:
- Add dried thyme, smoked paprika, ground cumin, ground coriander, and chopped garlic. Once fragrant, stir and simmer for one to two minutes.

Combine Tomatoes and Lentils:
- Fill the saucepan with diced tomatoes, veggie broth, bay leaf, and washed lentils. Add pepper and salt for seasoning.

Simmer:
- After bringing the mixture to a boil, lower the heat to a simmer, cover it, and cook the lentils for 25 to 30 minutes, or until they are soft.

Add the leafy greens:
- Cook the greens for a further five minutes, or until they have wilted, after stirring in the chopped spinach or kale.

Modify Seasoning:
- Use your taste buds to determine how much salt and pepper to add.

Finishing touches and serving:
- Take out the bay leaf. Pour the Lentil and Vegetable Stew into individual dishes and sprinkle with parsley, if desired.

Serve:

- You may alternatively serve the warm lentil and vegetable stew with a piece of crusty bread.

9. Spinach and Feta Stuffed Chicken

Ingredients:

- 4 boneless, skinless chicken breasts
- Salt and black pepper to taste
- 2 cups fresh spinach, chopped
- ½ cup crumbled feta cheese
- ¼ cup sun-dried tomatoes, chopped
- 2 cloves garlic, minced
- 1 tablespoon olive oil
- 1 teaspoon dried oregano
- 1 teaspoon dried basil
- 1 teaspoon paprika
- Toothpicks or kitchen twine for securing

Instructions:

Oven Prep:
 - Set the oven's temperature to 375°F, or 190°C.

 - Prepare the chicken by laying each breast flat and seasoning it with black pepper and salt on both sides.

Prepare Filling:
 - Heat olive oil in a pan over medium heat. When aromatic, add the minced garlic and sauté it.
 - Cook the chopped spinach until it wilts. Take off the heat.
 - Add the chopped sun-dried tomatoes, crumbled feta cheese, sautéed spinach, dried oregano, dried basil, and paprika to a bowl. Blend well.

Make a Pocket in the Chicken:
- Without cutting all the way through, make a horizontal slit down the side of each chicken breast.

Stuff Chicken:
- Stuff the spinach and feta mixture into each pocket of the chicken breast.

Secure with Toothpicks or Twine:
- If toothpicks are being used, use them to secure the aperture. Tie the packed chicken breast with string, if needed, to ensure the stuffing stays in place.

Season Exterior:
- Add a little more salt, black pepper, and paprika to the exterior of each packed chicken breast.

Sear the chicken:
- Heat a small amount of olive oil in an oven-safe pan over medium-high heat. Sear

the filled chicken breasts until golden brown, 2 to 3 minutes per side.

- Bake the chicken for 20 to 25 minutes, or until it is cooked through and reaches an internal temperature of 165°F (74°C), after transferring the skillet to the preheated oven.

Rest and Serve:
- Before serving, let the spinach and feta stuffed chicken sit for a few minutes.

Present:
- Present the packed chicken breasts at room temperature, with the option to top them off with more fresh herbs.

10. Pesto Pasta with Cherry Tomatoes

Ingredients:

- 8 oz (225g) pasta of your choice
- 1 cup fresh basil leaves, packed
- ½ cup grated Parmesan cheese
- ⅓ cup pine nuts
- 2 cloves garlic, peeled
- ½ cup extra-virgin olive oil
- Salt and black pepper to taste
- 1 cup cherry tomatoes, halved
- ¼ cup grated Pecorino Romano cheese (optional)
- Fresh basil leaves for garnish

Instructions:

- Cook the pasta in a large pot of salted boiling water until al dente, following the directions on the box. After draining, set away.

- To make pesto, pulse fresh basil, grated Parmesan cheese, pine nuts, and peeled garlic cloves in a food processor. Pulse until chopped finely. Olive oil should be added gradually while the food processor is operating in order to create a smooth pesto sauce. To taste, add salt and black pepper for seasoning.

Mix Pasta and Pesto:
 - Place the cooked pasta in a big bowl and toss to cover it thoroughly with the prepared pesto.

Add Cherry Tomatoes:
- Gently fold in the cherry tomatoes, halving them as you go to make sure they are all over the spaghetti.

Adjust Seasoning:
    - Taste and make any necessary adjustments by adding additional salt or pepper.

Optionally, add grated Pecorino Romano:

- To add even more flavor to the pesto pasta, feel free to sprinkle grated Pecorino Romano cheese on top.

Garnish and Serve:

- Sprinkle fresh basil leaves over the pesto pasta with cherry tomatoes.

Soup Recipes

1. Chicken Noodle Soup

Ingredients:

- 1 tablespoon olive oil
- 1 onion, finely chopped
- 2 carrots, sliced
- 2 celery stalks, sliced
- 3 cloves garlic, minced
- 1 teaspoon dried thyme
- 1 teaspoon dried rosemary
- 8 cups chicken broth
- 2 boneless, skinless chicken breasts
- Salt and black pepper to taste
- 8 oz (225g) egg noodles
- 1 cup frozen peas
- 2 tablespoons fresh parsley, chopped
- Lemon wedges for serving (optional)

Instructions:

Sauté Vegetables:
 - Place a big saucepan over medium heat with olive oil. Add the sliced carrots, sliced celery, and finely chopped onion. Sauté the veggies till they get tender.

Add Aromatics:
 - Add dried rosemary, dry thyme, and chopped garlic. Cook, stirring, for a further one to two minutes, or until aromatic.

Add Chicken Broth:
 - Add the chicken broth and raise the temperature until it boils.

Prepare the chicken:
 - Place the skinless, boneless chicken breasts in the saucepan. Put some salt and black pepper over it. Simmer until the chicken is well cooked, 15 to 20 minutes.

Take Out and Shred the Chicken:
- Take out the chicken breasts from the saucepan. Using two forks, shred the chicken and add it back to the soup.

Cook Egg Noodles:
- Place the egg noodles in the saucepan and cook them until they are al dente, following the directions on the package.

Add Frozen Peas:
- Add frozen peas to the noodles in the final few minutes of cooking. They'll cook fast.

Adjust Seasoning:
- If necessary, add additional salt and black pepper to the soup after tasting it.

Garnish with Parsley:
- Just before serving, stir in freshly cut parsley.

- To serve, spoon the chicken noodle soup into individual bowls. Serve with lemon wedges on the side for a welcome burst of citrus.

2. Butternut Squash Soup

Ingredients:

- 1 large butternut squash, peeled, seeded, and diced (about 4 cups)
- 1 onion, chopped
- 2 carrots, peeled and chopped
- 2 apples, peeled, cored, and chopped
- 3 cloves garlic, minced
- 1 teaspoon ground cinnamon
- ½ teaspoon ground nutmeg
- ½ teaspoon ground ginger
- 4 cups vegetable broth
- 1 cup coconut milk
- 2 tablespoons olive oil
- Salt and black pepper to taste
- Pumpkin seeds and fresh parsley for garnish (optional)

Instructions:

Oven Prep:
 - Set the oven's temperature to 400°F, or 200°C.

 - To roast butternut squash, place it in diced form on a baking sheet. Add a drizzle of olive oil and season with black pepper and salt. Roast the squash for 30 to 35 minutes, or until it's soft and beginning to caramelize.

Sauté the Vegetables:
 - Heat the olive oil in a big saucepan over medium heat. Add the diced apples, carrots, and onion. Sauté the veggies till they get tender.

Add Aromatics:
 - Add ground ginger, ground nutmeg, ground cinnamon, and chopped garlic. Cook, stirring, for a further one to two minutes, or until aromatic.

Mix Roasted Squash:
- Include the roasted butternut squash in the saucepan and toss it in with the veggies that have been sautéed.

Add veggie Broth:
- Add the veggie broth and boil the mixture. Simmer for 15 to 20 minutes to let the flavors combine.

Blend Soup:
- Pour the soup into a blender in batches or use an immersion blender. Blend till creamy and smooth.

Add Coconut Milk:
- To create a rich, velvety texture, stir in coconut milk. Simmer for five more minutes.

Modify Seasoning:
- Taste the soup and add more salt and black pepper if necessary.

Add garnish and serve:

- Spoon butternut squash soup into individual bowls. If preferred, garnish with fresh parsley and pumpkin seeds.

3. Tomato Basil Soup

Ingredients:

- 2 tablespoons olive oil
- 1 onion, chopped
- 2 carrots, peeled and chopped
- 3 cloves garlic, minced
- 2 cans (28 oz each) whole tomatoes, undrained
- 1 can (14 oz) diced tomatoes, undrained
- 4 cups vegetable broth
- 1 teaspoon sugar
- 1 teaspoon dried basil
- ½ teaspoon dried oregano
- Salt and black pepper to taste

- ½ cup heavy cream or coconut milk (optional)
- Fresh basil leaves for garnish

Instructions:

Sauté Vegetables:
 - Place a big saucepan over medium heat with olive oil. Add the carrots and onion, chopped. Sauté the veggies till they get tender.

Add Garlic:
 - Cook the minced garlic for a further one to two minutes, or until it becomes aromatic.

Add the tomatoes:
 - Add the chopped and whole tomatoes, together with their liquids. Using a spoon, break up the entire tomatoes.

Pour the Vegetable Broth:
- Include the sugar, dried oregano and basil, and the vegetable broth. Put some salt and black pepper over it.

Simmer:
- Simmer the soup for a short while. To allow the flavors to mingle, simmer it for 20 to 25 minutes.

Blend Soup:
- Blend the soup until it's smooth using an immersion blender. Or, pour the soup in batches into a blender, puree, and then pour back into the saucepan.

Add Cream (Optional):
- If used, stir in coconut milk or heavy cream. Simmer for five more minutes.

Modify Seasoning:
- Taste the soup and add more salt and black pepper if necessary.

Finish and Present:

- Spoon the Tomato Basil Soup into individual bowls. Add some fresh basil leaves as garnish.

Serve:

- If preferred, serve the soup warm with croutons or crusty toast.

4. Minestrone Soup

Ingredients:

- 2 tablespoons olive oil
- 1 onion, chopped
- 2 carrots, diced
- 2 celery stalks, diced
- 3 cloves garlic, minced
- 1 zucchini, diced
- 1 yellow squash, diced
- 1 cup green beans, chopped
- 1 can (14 oz) diced tomatoes, undrained

- 1 can (15 oz) kidney beans, drained and rinsed
- 1 can (15 oz) cannellini beans, drained and rinsed
- 8 cups vegetable broth
- 1 teaspoon dried oregano
- 1 teaspoon dried basil
- ½ teaspoon dried thyme
- 1 cup small pasta (such as ditalini or small shells)
- Salt and black pepper to taste
- 2 cups fresh spinach or kale, chopped
- Grated Parmesan cheese for serving (optional)

Instructions:

Sauté Vegetables:
- Place a big saucepan over medium heat with olive oil. Add the minced garlic, diced celery, diced carrots, and sliced onion. Sauté the veggies till they get tender.

Add Zucchini, Yellow Squash, and Green Beans:

- Fill the saucepan with chopped green beans, diced zucchini, and diced yellow squash. Simmer for five more minutes.

Add the Beans and Tomatoes:

- Add the chopped tomatoes together with their liquids. Add the washed and drained cannellini and kidney beans. Mix thoroughly.

Pour the Vegetable stock:

- Include the dried thyme, dried basil, and dried oregano in the vegetable stock. Put some salt and black pepper over it.

Simmer:

- Simmer the soup for a short while. Let it simmer for fifteen to twenty minutes so that the flavors may combine.

Cook Pasta:
- Place tiny pasta in the saucepan and cook until al dente, following the directions on the package.

Add Leafy Greens:
- In the final few minutes of cooking, stir in finely chopped fresh spinach or kale until it wilts.

Adjust Seasoning:
- Use salt and black pepper to taste the minestrone soup and make any necessary adjustments.

- To serve, spoon soup into individual dishes. Before serving, feel free to sprinkle some grated Parmesan cheese on top.

5. Lentil Soup

Ingredients:

- 1 cup dry green or brown lentils, rinsed and drained
- 2 tablespoons olive oil
- 1 onion, finely chopped
- 2 carrots, diced
- 2 celery stalks, diced
- 3 cloves garlic, minced
- 1 teaspoon ground cumin
- 1 teaspoon ground coriander
- ½ teaspoon smoked paprika
- ½ teaspoon dried thyme
- 6 cups vegetable broth
- 1 can (14 oz) diced tomatoes, undrained
- Salt and black pepper to taste
- Juice of 1 lemon
- Fresh parsley for garnish

Instructions:

 - To prepare the lentils, rinse them in cold water and then drain them.

Sauté Vegetables:
 - Place a large saucepan over medium heat with olive oil. Add diced celery, diced carrots, and chopped onion. Sauté the veggies till they get tender.

Add the Spices and Garlic:
- Add the dried thyme, smoked paprika, ground cumin, ground coriander, and minced garlic. Cook, stirring, for a further one to two minutes, or until aromatic.

Combine Lentils and Tomatoes:
 - Fill the saucepan with chopped tomatoes and their liquids after the lentils have been washed. Mix thoroughly.

Add the Vegetable Broth:
 - Add the vegetable broth and heat the mixture until it boils. Once the lentils are soft, reduce heat to low, cover, and simmer for 25 to 30 minutes.

Add Lemon Juice and Season:
- Toss in the lentil soup and season with salt and black pepper to taste. Add one lemon's juice to the soup and mix it in.

Adjust Seasoning:
 - Taste the soup and make any necessary adjustments by adding extra salt, pepper, or lemon juice.

Garnish and Serve:
 - Spoon Lentil Soup into individual dishes. Add fresh parsley as a garnish.

6. Creamy Broccoli Cheddar Soup

Ingredients:

- 4 cups fresh broccoli florets
- 1 onion, chopped
- 2 carrots, peeled and diced
- 2 celery stalks, diced
- 3 tablespoons unsalted butter
- ¼ cup all-purpose flour
- 4 cups vegetable or chicken broth
- 2 cups whole milk
- 2 cups shredded sharp cheddar cheese
- Salt and black pepper to taste
- ½ teaspoon dried mustard (optional)
- ¼ teaspoon nutmeg (optional)
- Croutons and additional shredded cheddar
for garnish (optional)

Instructions:

Assemble the vegetables:
- Chop the fresh broccoli into tiny pieces. Dice the celery and carrots, and chop the onion.

Sauté Vegetables:
- Melt butter in a large saucepan over medium heat. Add diced celery, diced carrots, and chopped onion. Sauté the veggies till they get tender.

Add Flour:
- Dredge the sautéed veggies in all-purpose flour. To make a roux, stir constantly for two to three minutes.

Pour Milk and Broth:
- Stir continuously to prevent lumps as you gradually add the chicken or veggie broth. Stir with whole milk after adding it.

Simmer:
- Cook the mixture for ten to fifteen minutes, or until the veggies are soft, by bringing it to a simmer.

- Toss in the broccoli florets and boil for a further five to seven minutes, or until the broccoli is tender but retains its bright green color.

Blend Soup (Optional):
- Blend some of the soup with an immersion blender to give it a creamier texture. Or, put some of it in a blender and puree it, then put it back in the saucepan.

Add the Sharp Cheddar Cheese:
- Add the shredded cheese and stir until it melts and becomes smooth.

Season:
- Add salt, black pepper, nutmeg (optional), and dry mustard to the soup. To suit your taste, adjust.

Garnish and Serve:
 - Spoon the Cheddar-Cream Broccoli Soup into individual bowls. Garnish with more shredded cheddar and croutons, if desired.

7. Spicy Black Bean Soup

Ingredients:

- 2 cans (15 oz each) black beans, drained and rinsed
- 1 onion, chopped
- 2 bell peppers (any color), diced
- 2 jalapeños, seeded and finely chopped
- 3 cloves garlic, minced
- 1 teaspoon ground cumin
- 1 teaspoon chili powder
- ½ teaspoon smoked paprika
- 4 cups vegetable broth
- 1 can (14 oz) diced tomatoes, undrained
- 1 cup corn kernels (fresh or frozen)
- Juice of 2 limes

- Salt and black pepper to taste
- Fresh cilantro for garnish
- Sour cream or Greek yogurt for topping (optional)

Instructions:

- To prepare the vegetables, finely cut the jalapeños, dice the bell peppers, chop the onion, and mince the garlic.

Sauté Vegetables:
- In a big saucepan, soften the diced bell peppers, jalapeños, and onion by sautéing them.

Add the Spices and Garlic:
- Add the smoked paprika, ground cumin, chili powder, and chopped garlic. Cook, stirring, for a further one to two minutes, or until aromatic.

Combine Tomatoes and Black Beans:
ok - Fill the saucepan with diced tomatoes, their juices, and vegetable broth after the black beans have been drained and washed. Mix thoroughly.

Simmer:
- To let the flavors mingle, bring the soup to a simmer and cook for 15 to 20 minutes.

- Add Corn, simmer for a further five minutes after stirring in frozen or fresh corn kernels.

- Pour the soup with the juice of two limes. Mix thoroughly.

- Add salt and black pepper to taste when preparing the spicy black bean soup. As necessary, adjust the seasoning.

- Spoon soup into individual dishes. Add fresh cilantro as a garnish.

- You can choose to add a dollop of Greek yogurt or sour cream on the top of each dish.

8. Chicken and Vegetable Stir-Fry with Tofu

Ingredients:

- 1 lb (450g) firm tofu, pressed and cubed
- 2 tablespoons soy sauce
- 2 tablespoons hoisin sauce
- 1 tablespoon sesame oil
- 2 tablespoons vegetable oil, divided
- 1 lb (450g) boneless, skinless chicken breast, thinly sliced
- 3 cups broccoli florets
- 1 bell pepper, thinly sliced
- 2 carrots, julienned
- 3 cloves garlic, minced
- 1 tablespoon fresh ginger, grated
- 2 green onions, sliced
- Cooked brown rice or quinoa for serving

Instructions:

- To marinate tofu, place cubed tofu, hoisin sauce, soy sauce, and sesame oil in a bowl. Let the tofu marinate for at least fifteen minutes, gently tossing to coat.

Sauté Tofu:
- Heat 1 tablespoon of vegetable oil over medium-high heat in a large wok or pan. When the tofu has marinated, add it and fry it till golden brown all over. Take out of the wok and place aside.

Cook the chicken:
- Add the final tablespoon of vegetable oil to the same pan. Cook the chicken slices until they are well done and browned. Take out of the wok and place aside.

Stir-Fry Vegetables:
- Fill the wok with bell pepper, carrots, and broccoli that have been finely chopped.

Stir-fry the veggies for 3–4 minutes, or until they are crisp-tender.

Add Aromatics:
 - Move the veggies to one side of the wok and stir in the grated ginger and minced garlic. Sauté until aromatic, one to two minutes.

Combine Chicken, Tofu, and Vegetables:
 - Add the cooked chicken and tofu back to the skillet and toss everything together.

Conclude and Add Garnish:
 - Add the sliced green onions and simmer for a minute more. Make sure the sauce coats everything well.

 - To serve, arrange the cooked brown rice or quinoa on top of the Chicken and Vegetable Stir-Fry with Tofu.

9. Mushroom Barley Soup

Ingredients:

- 1 cup pearl barley, rinsed and drained
- 2 tablespoons olive oil
- 1 onion, finely chopped
- 2 carrots, diced
- 2 celery stalks, diced
- 3 cloves garlic, minced
- 8 oz (225g) mushrooms, sliced
- 1 teaspoon dried thyme
- 1 teaspoon dried rosemary
- 8 cups vegetable broth
- 1 bay leaf
- Salt and black pepper to taste
- Fresh parsley for garnish

Instructions:

- To prepare barley, follow the directions on the package and simmer it in a small pot. After cooking, place aside.

Sauté Vegetables:
- Place a large saucepan over medium heat with olive oil. Add diced celery, diced carrots, and chopped onion. Sauté the veggies till they get tender.

Add Mushrooms and Garlic:
- Add sliced mushrooms and minced garlic. Simmer the mushrooms for a further five to seven minutes, or until they start to dry up and turn golden brown.

Add Herbs to Season:
- Mix in the dried rosemary and thyme. Cook the herbs for a further one to two minutes, or until aromatic.

Pour Vegetable Broth:
- Add a bay leaf and pour in the vegetable broth. Simmer the soup for a while.

Simmer:

- To enable the flavors to mingle, simmer the mushroom-barley soup for 20 to 25 minutes.

Add Cooked Barley:

- Fill the saucepan with the cooked pearl barley. Mix well to blend.

Modify Seasoning:

- Add salt and black pepper to taste when preparing the soup. As necessary, adjust the seasoning.

Finishing Touches and Serving:

- Take out the bay leaf. Spoon the Barley Soup into individual bowls. Add fresh parsley as a garnish.

10. Coconut Curry Cauliflower Soup

Ingredients:

- 1 head cauliflower, chopped into florets
- 2 tablespoons coconut oil
- 1 onion, chopped
- 3 cloves garlic, minced
- 1 tablespoon ginger, grated
- 2 tablespoons curry powder
- 1 teaspoon ground turmeric
- 1 can (14 oz) coconut milk
- 4 cups vegetable broth
- Salt and black pepper to taste
- Juice of 1 lime
- Fresh cilantro for garnish
- Toasted coconut flakes for topping (optional)

Instructions:

- Before roasting the cauliflower, preheat the oven to 400°F, or 200°C. Spread the cauliflower florets out on a baking sheet after tossing them with one tablespoon of coconut oil. Roast for 20 to 25 minutes, or until soft and golden brown.

Sauté Aromatics:
- Heat the remaining 1 tablespoon of coconut oil in a big saucepan. Add the grated ginger, minced garlic, and chopped onion. The onion should be sautéed until transparent.

Add Curry and Turmeric:
- Cook for a further one to two minutes, or until aromatic, after stirring in the curry powder and crushed turmeric.

- Toss the roasted cauliflower into the saucepan to coat it with the fragrant mixture. 4. Combine Roasted Cauliflower.

Pour in Vegetable Broth and Coconut Milk:
- Pour in the vegetable broth and coconut milk. Simmer the soup for a while.

Simmer:
- To enable the flavors to blend, simmer the Coconut Curry Cauliflower Soup for 15 to 20 minutes.

Blend Soup:
- Puree the soup in a blender or with an immersion blender until it's smooth.

Adjust Seasoning and Add Lime Juice:
- Taste and adjust the soup's seasoning with salt and black pepper. Stir the soup after adding one lime's juice.

Garnish and Serve:
- Spoon soup into individual dishes. Add some fresh cilantro and toasted coconut flakes, if preferred, as garnish.

Chapter 10

Main Course Recipes

Omnivore Main Recipes:

1. Grilled Lemon Herb Chicken

Ingredients:

- 4 boneless, skinless chicken breasts
- ¼ cup olive oil
- 2 tablespoons fresh lemon juice
- 2 cloves garlic, minced
- 1 teaspoon dried oregano
- 1 teaspoon dried thyme
- 1 teaspoon dried rosemary
- 1 teaspoon paprika
- Salt and black pepper to taste
- Lemon slices for garnish (optional)
- Fresh parsley for garnish (optional)

Instructions:

- To marinate chicken, combine olive oil, fresh lemon juice, minced garlic, dried thyme, dried rosemary, dried oregano, paprika, salt, and black pepper in a bowl.

- Prepare the chicken breasts by putting them in a shallow dish or resealable plastic bag. Make sure the chicken is well covered by pouring the marinade over it. Allow to marinate for a minimum of half an hour and a maximum of four hours.

Preheat the Grill:
- Turn the heat up to medium-high.

Grill the chicken:
- Take it out of the marinade and let any extra to fall off. The chicken should be cooked through after 6 to 8 minutes on each side of the grill. A temperature of 165°F (74°C) should be reached inside.

- Let the grilled lemon herb chicken rest for a few minutes after removing it from the grill. Then, garnish it. If preferred, garnish with fresh parsley and lemon slices.

Serve:
- Accompany the Grilled Lemon Herb Chicken with your preferred side dishes, including rice, a crisp salad, or grilled veggies.

2. Baked Salmon with Dill Sauce

Ingredients:

For Baked Salmon:
- 4 salmon filets
- 2 tablespoons olive oil
- 2 tablespoons lemon juice
- 2 cloves garlic, minced
- 1 teaspoon dried dill
- Salt and black pepper to taste
- Lemon slices for garnish (optional)
- Fresh dill for garnish (optional)

For Dill Sauce:
- ½ cup Greek yogurt
- 1 tablespoon mayonnaise
- 1 tablespoon fresh dill, chopped
- 1 teaspoon Dijon mustard
- 1 teaspoon lemon juice
- Salt and black pepper to taste

Instructions:

- For the salmon, marinate: Mix the olive oil, lemon juice, dried dill, minced garlic, salt, and black pepper in a bowl. Pour the marinade over the salmon filets and place them in a shallow dish. In the fridge, let them marinade for at least half an hour.

Preheat Oven:
- Set the oven's temperature to 200°C, or 400°F.

Bake the Salmon:
- Arrange the marinated filets on a parchment paper-lined baking sheet. Bake

for 12 to 15 minutes, or until a fork can easily pierce the salmon, in a preheated oven.

Prepare the Dill Sauce:
- Combine the Greek yogurt, mayonnaise, Dijon mustard, chopped fresh dill, lemon juice, salt, and black pepper in a small dish. Mix well until fully incorporated.

- To serve, remove the salmon filets from the oven and place them on serving plates. Pour dill sauce over each filet.

- If preferred, add fresh dill and lemon slices as garnish.

- Pair the baked salmon with dill sauce with your preferred side dishes, including quinoa or roasted veggies.

3. Beef Stir-Fry with Vegetables

Ingredients:

- 1 lb (450g) beef sirloin or flank steak, thinly sliced
- 3 tablespoons soy sauce
- 2 tablespoons oyster sauce
- 1 tablespoon hoisin sauce
- 1 tablespoon sesame oil
- 2 tablespoons vegetable oil, divided
- 3 cloves garlic, minced
- 1 tablespoon ginger, grated
- 1 broccoli crown, cut into florets
- 1 bell pepper, thinly sliced
- 1 carrot, julienned
- 1 cup snap peas, ends trimmed
- 2 green onions, sliced
- Cooked rice or noodles for serving

Instructions:

- Marinate the meat by combining the thinly sliced steak, hoisin sauce, oyster sauce, and sesame oil in a dish. Give it a minimum of fifteen minutes to marinate.

Prepare the Vegetables:
- Slice the bell pepper thinly, chop the carrot into julienne pieces, and trim the snap peas.

Heat pan or Wok:
- In a large pan or wok, heat 1 tablespoon of vegetable oil over high heat.

Sear Beef:
- Quickly stir-fry the marinated beef in the heated wok until it is browned and well done. After taking the steak out of the pan, set it aside.

- To sauté aromatics, add the last tablespoon of vegetable oil to the same pan. Add the grated ginger and minced garlic. Sauté until aromatic, approximately 30 seconds.

Stir-Fry Vegetables:
 - Fill the wok with bell pepper, broccoli, julienned carrot, and snap peas. Stir-fry the veggies for 3–4 minutes, or until they are crisp-tender.

Mix meat and Vegetables:
 - Add the cooked meat back to the pan and mix everything thoroughly.

Conclude and Add Garnish:
 - Add the sliced green onions and simmer for a minute more. Make sure the sauce coats everything well.

 - To serve, arrange the Beef Stir-Fry with Vegetables on top of prepared noodles or rice.

4. Pesto Shrimp Pasta

Ingredients:

- 8 oz (225g) linguine or your preferred pasta
- 1 lb (450g) large shrimp, peeled and deveined
- 2 tablespoons olive oil
- 3 cloves garlic, minced
- ½ cup cherry tomatoes, halved
- ⅓ cup store-bought or homemade pesto sauce
- Salt and black pepper to taste
- Red pepper flakes (optional for added heat)
- Fresh basil leaves for garnish
- Grated Parmesan cheese for serving

Instructions:

Cook Pasta:
  - Cook the pasta until al dente, following the directions on the package. Before

draining, set aside roughly 1/2 cup of pasta water.

Sauté Shrimp:

- Heat olive oil in a big pan over medium-high heat. When the shrimp are pink and opaque, add the minced garlic and sauté for two to three minutes on each side.

Add Tomatoes:

- Add the cherry tomatoes, cut in half, to the pan and simmer for a further one to two minutes, or until the tomatoes begin to soften.

Combine Pesto:

- Make sure the shrimp and tomatoes are thoroughly coated by stirring in the pesto sauce. To get the right consistency, thin down any excess sauce by adding a little amount of the pasta water that was set aside.

- Add salt and black pepper to taste when preparing the pesto shrimp pasta. If you enjoy a little spice, add some red pepper flakes.

- Transfer the cooked and drained pasta into the frying pan. Make sure the pasta is well covered in the pesto sauce by tossing everything together.

- Arrange the Pesto Shrimp Pasta into dishes and top with freshly grated Parmesan cheese and basil leaves.

5. Honey Mustard Glazed Pork Chops

Ingredients:

- 4 bone-in pork chops
- ¼ cup Dijon mustard
- 2 tablespoons honey
- 1 tablespoon whole grain mustard
- 2 cloves garlic, minced
- 1 tablespoon soy sauce

- 1 tablespoon olive oil
- Salt and black pepper to taste
- Fresh parsley for garnish

Instructions:

Oven Prep:
 - Set the oven's temperature to 375°F, or 190°C.

Season Pork Chops:
 - Use black pepper and salt to season the pork chops.

 - Prepare the Honey Mustard Glaze by whisking together the Dijon mustard, honey, whole grain mustard, olive oil, soy sauce, and chopped garlic in a bowl.

Glaze Pork Chops:
 - Make sure the pork chops are well covered by brushing them with the honey mustard glaze.

- Transfer the pork chops with glaze to a baking tray. Bake until the internal temperature reaches 145°F (63°C), about 25 to 30 minutes.

- Sprinkle the Honey Mustard Glazed Pork Chops with freshly chopped parsley and serve them hot.

6. Lemon Butter Garlic Shrimp

Ingredients:

- 1 lb (450g) large shrimp, peeled and deveined
- 3 tablespoons butter
- 3 cloves garlic, minced
- Zest of 1 lemon
- Juice of 1 lemon
- 1 tablespoon fresh parsley, chopped
- Salt and black pepper to taste
- Red pepper flakes (optional for added heat)

Instructions:

-    Shrimp should be sautéed by melting butter in a pan over medium heat. When aromatic, add the minced garlic and sauté it.

Cook Shrimp:
- Place the shrimp in the skillet and cook them for two to three minutes on each side, or until they become opaque and pink.

Add Lemon Zest and Juice:
- Make sure the shrimp are thoroughly covered by stirring in the lemon zest and lemon juice.

- Add salt, black pepper, and red pepper flakes, if preferred, to the Lemon Butter Garlic Shrimp. To allow the flavors to mingle, cook for one more minute.

- Add freshly cut parsley as a garnish. Serve the shrimp warm on crusty bread or over rice.

7. Teriyaki Chicken Skewers

Ingredients:

- 1 lb (450g) boneless, skinless chicken thighs, cut into bite-sized pieces
- ½ cup soy sauce
- ¼ cup mirin (Japanese sweet rice wine)
- 2 tablespoons honey
- 1 tablespoon rice vinegar
- 2 cloves garlic, minced
- 1 teaspoon ginger, grated
- 1 tablespoon cornstarch
- 1 tablespoon water
- Sesame seeds and sliced green onions for garnish (optional)

Instructions:

Marinate the chicken:
 - To make the teriyaki marinade, mix the soy sauce, mirin, honey, rice vinegar, chopped garlic, and grated ginger in a basin.

Make sure the chicken pieces are well covered by placing them in the marinade. Place it in the fridge to marinate for at least half an hour.

Preheat Oven or Grill:
 - Turn the heat up to medium-high on your oven or grill.

 - Get the skewers ready by putting the marinated chicken pieces on them. To avoid burning, soak wooden skewers in water for approximately half an hour before using.

 - To prepare Teriyaki Sauce, mix cornstarch and water into a slurry in a small pot. Pour the saucepan's leftover marinade from the basin. Stir continuously while heating over medium heat until the sauce thickens. Take off the heat.

 - Grill the chicken skewers until they are cooked through, about 5 to 7 minutes each side. Last few minutes of grilling: baste the skewers with the thickened teriyaki sauce.

- If preferred, top the Teriyaki Chicken Skewers with sliced green onions and sesame seeds after they've cooked.

- You may serve the skewers with your preferred side dishes or over a bed of steaming rice. Any leftover teriyaki sauce should be drizzled on top.

8. Lamb Chops with Mint Pesto

Ingredients:

For Lamb Chops:
- 8 lamb chops
- 2 tablespoons olive oil
- 3 cloves garlic, minced
- 1 teaspoon dried rosemary
- Salt and black pepper to taste

For Mint Pesto:

- 1 cup fresh mint leaves
- ½ cup fresh basil leaves
- ⅓ cup pine nuts, toasted
- ½ cup Parmesan cheese, grated
- 2 cloves garlic
- ½ cup extra-virgin olive oil
- Salt and black pepper to taste
- Juice of 1 lemon

Instructions:

- To marinate lamb chops, combine olive oil, salt, black pepper, chopped garlic, and dried rosemary in a basin. Apply this mixture to the lamb chops and let them marinade for a minimum of half an hour.

- Prepare the grill for medium-high heat before grilling the lamb chops. Lamb chops should be cooked on the grill for 4–5 minutes on each side, or until done to your preference.

Get the mint pesto ready:
 - Mint, basil, roasted pine nuts, Parmesan cheese, garlic, and lemon juice should all be combined in a food processor. Pulse until thoroughly mixed. Olive oil should be added gradually while the machine is operating, until the pesto has a smooth consistency. To taste, add salt and black pepper for seasoning.

Serve:
 - Serve grilled lamb chops with a generous dollop of mint pesto on top.

9. Chicken Alfredo with Broccoli

Ingredients:

- 8 oz (225g) fettuccine pasta
- 2 tablespoons butter
- 2 boneless, skinless chicken breasts, thinly sliced
- 3 cloves garlic, minced
- 1 cup broccoli florets

- 1 cup heavy cream
- 1 cup Parmesan cheese, grated
- Salt and black pepper to taste
- Fresh parsley for garnish

Instructions:

Prepare Pasta:
- Follow the directions on the package to cook the fettuccine pasta. After draining, set away.

Sauté the chicken and broccoli:
- Melt the butter in a big pan over medium-high heat. Cook the chicken slices till they are browned. When the broccoli is crisp-tender, add the minced garlic and the broccoli florets and sauté.

- Prepare the Alfredo sauce by adding the heavy cream and simmering it. Once the sauce is creamy, turn down the heat and whisk in the grated Parmesan cheese. To taste, add salt and black pepper for seasoning.

- Toss the cooked fettuccine pasta in the skillet to cover it with the Alfredo sauce. 4. Combine Pasta and Sauce.

- Sprinkle the Chicken Alfredo with Broccoli with freshly cut parsley and serve hot.

10. Spicy BBQ Ribs

Ingredients:

- 2 racks baby back ribs
- 1 cup BBQ sauce
- ¼ cup apple cider vinegar
- 2 tablespoons brown sugar
- 1 tablespoon paprika
- 1 teaspoon garlic powder
- 1 teaspoon onion powder
- 1 teaspoon cayenne pepper
- Salt and black pepper to taste

Instructions:

- To prepare the ribs, first peel off the membrane covering the back of each rib. Put some salt and black pepper over it.

Prepare the BBQ Sauce:
- Combine the BBQ sauce, brown sugar, onion powder, garlic powder, cayenne pepper, and apple cider vinegar in a bowl.

Marinate and Grill Ribs:
- Reserving part of the BBQ sauce mixture for basting, coat the ribs with it. Let it marinate for two hours or overnight. Set the grill's temperature to medium. Baste the ribs with the saved sauce while you grill them for 20 to 30 minutes on each side.

Serve:
- Cut and serve the spicy barbecue ribs hot once they are well cooked and caramelized.

Vegetarian Main Recipes:

1. Vegetarian Eggplant Lasagna

Ingredients:

- 1 large eggplant, thinly sliced lengthwise
- 2 cups marinara sauce
- 1 cup ricotta cheese
- 1 cup mozzarella cheese, shredded
- ½ cup Parmesan cheese, grated
- 1 egg
- 2 cloves garlic, minced
- 1 teaspoon dried oregano
- Salt and black pepper to taste
- Fresh basil for garnish

Instructions:

Preheat Oven:
   - Turn the oven on to 375°F, or 190°C.

Grill Eggplant:

- To soften eggplant slices, brush them with olive oil and grill or roast them.

Prepare Filling:
- Combine ricotta cheese, dried oregano, minced garlic, half of the mozzarella, half of the Parmesan, beaten egg, salt, and black pepper in a bowl.

Assemble Lasagna:
- Arrange the grilled eggplant pieces, ricotta filling, and marinara sauce in a baking dish. Continue layering, and then cover with a layer of marinara sauce. Top with the remaining Parmesan and mozzarella.

Bake:
- The vegetarian eggplant lasagna should be baked for 25 to 30 minutes, or until the cheese is bubbling and melted.

Garnish and Serve:
- Sprinkle the lasagna with freshly chopped basil and serve it hot.

2. Chickpea and Spinach Curry

Ingredients:

- 2 cans (15 oz each) chickpeas, drained and
rinsed
- 1 onion, finely chopped
- 3 tomatoes, chopped
- 2 cups fresh spinach
- 2 cloves garlic, minced
- 1 tablespoon ginger, grated
- 1 can (14 oz) coconut milk
- 2 tablespoons curry powder
- 1 teaspoon cumin
- 1 teaspoon turmeric
- Salt and red pepper flakes to taste
- Fresh cilantro for garnish

Instructions:

Sauté Aromatics:
 - Using a big pot, add the minced garlic, grated ginger, chopped onion and sauté until aromatic.

Add Spices:
 - Mix in turmeric, cumin, and curry powder. Simmer for one more minute.

Cook the Chickpeas:
 - Include the diced tomatoes and chickpeas in the saucepan. Cook until the tomatoes are tender, 5 to 7 minutes.

Add Coconut Milk:
 - Add the coconut milk and cook the curry. Add some salt and crushed red pepper to taste.

Include Spinach:
 - Include fresh spinach in the saucepan and let it wilt.

Garnish and Serve:

 - Sprinkle some fresh cilantro over the chickpea and spinach curry. Serve it over naan or over rice.

3. Mushroom and Spinach Stuffed Bell Peppers

Ingredients:

- 4 large bell peppers, halved and seeds removed
- 2 cups mushrooms, finely chopped
- 2 cups fresh spinach, chopped
- 1 onion, finely chopped
- 2 cloves garlic, minced
- 1 cup quinoa, cooked
- 1 cup mozzarella cheese, shredded
- ½ cup Parmesan cheese, grated
- 2 tablespoons olive oil
- Salt and black pepper to taste

- Fresh parsley for garnish

Instructions:

Oven Prep:
 - Set the oven's temperature to 375°F, or 190°C.

Sauté Vegetables:
 - In a skillet, soften chopped onions, garlic, and mushrooms with olive oil. Cook the chopped spinach until it wilts.

Prepare Filling:
 - Combine cooked quinoa, mozzarella, Parmesan, and sautéed veggies in a bowl. Put some salt and black pepper over it.

Stuff Bell Peppers:
 - Stuff the veggie and quinoa mixture into each side of a bell pepper.

Bake:

- Transfer the stuffed bell peppers with spinach and mushrooms to a baking tray. Bake the peppers for 25 to 30 minutes, or until they are soft.

Garnish and Serve:
  - Sprinkle the filled bell peppers with freshly chopped parsley and serve them hot.

4. Caprese Stuffed Portobello Mushrooms

Ingredients:

- 4 large Portobello mushrooms, stems removed
- 1 cup cherry tomatoes, halved
- 1 cup fresh mozzarella balls, halved
- ¼ cup fresh basil, chopped
- 2 tablespoons balsamic glaze
- 2 tablespoons olive oil
- Salt and black pepper to taste

Instructions:

Preheat Oven:
   - Turn the oven on to 375°F, or 190°C.

Mushroom Preparation:
 - Wash and arrange Portobello mushrooms on a baking sheet.

Assemble the Caprese Filling:
 - Arrange cherry tomatoes, mozzarella balls, and finely chopped fresh basil into each mushroom.

Drizzle and Season:
 - Drizzle the packed mushrooms with olive oil. Put some salt and black pepper over it.

Bake:
 - Bake the stuffed portobello mushrooms with caprese for 15 to 20 minutes, or until the cheese has melted and the mushrooms are soft.

Sprinkle Balsamic Glaze:
- After taking the stuffed mushrooms out of the oven, sprinkle each one with balsamic glaze.

Present:
- Present the mushrooms warm, topped with more freshly chopped basil if preferred.

5. Vegetarian Thai Green Curry

Ingredients:

- 1 can (14 oz) coconut milk
- 2 tablespoons green curry paste
- 1 cup tofu, cubed
- 1 cup broccoli florets
- 1 red bell pepper, sliced
- 1 carrot, julienned
- 1 zucchini, sliced
- 1 cup snap peas, ends trimmed
- 1 tablespoon soy sauce
- 1 tablespoon brown sugar
- Fresh basil leaves for garnish

- Cooked rice for serving

Instructions:

Simmer Curry Paste and Coconut Milk:
- In a saucepan, thoroughly mix the green curry paste and coconut milk over medium heat.

Add Tofu and Vegetables:
- Fill the saucepan with cubed tofu, broccoli, red bell pepper, zucchini, and julienned carrots. Sauté the veggies until they are soft.

- Add seasoning by mixing in brown sugar and soy sauce. Taste and adjust the seasoning.

- To serve, place the cooked rice on top of the vegetarian Thai green curry and top with fresh basil leaves.

6. Quinoa Stuffed Acorn Squash

Ingredients:

- 2 acorn squash, halved and seeds removed
- 1 cup quinoa, cooked
- 1 cup black beans, cooked
- 1 cup corn kernels (fresh or frozen)
- 1 cup cherry tomatoes, halved
- ½ cup red onion, finely chopped
- ¼ cup cilantro, chopped
- Juice of 1 lime
- 2 tablespoons olive oil
- Salt and black pepper to taste
- Avocado slices for garnish (optional)

Instructions:

Preheat Oven:
    - Set oven temperature to 400°F, or 200°C.

Roast Acorn Squash:

- Arrange the halves of the squash on a baking sheet. Roast until they are soft, about 30 to 35 minutes.

Make the Quinoa Filling:

- Put the cooked quinoa, black beans, corn, avocado, red onion, cilantro, lime juice, and olive oil in a bowl. Blend well.

Season:

- Add salt and black pepper to taste when adding seasoning to the quinoa mixture.

Stuffed Acorn Squash:

- Spoon the quinoa mixture into each half of cooked acorn squash.

To serve:

- If preferred, garnish with avocado slices. Warm quinoa-stuffed acorn squash should be served.

7. Vegetarian Fajita Bowl

Ingredients:

For Fajita Vegetables:
- 1 red bell pepper, sliced
- 1 yellow bell pepper, sliced
- 1 green bell pepper, sliced
- 1 red onion, sliced
- 2 tablespoons olive oil
- 1 tablespoon fajita seasoning

For Black Beans:
- 1 can (15 oz) black beans, drained and rinsed
- 1 teaspoon cumin
- ½ teaspoon chili powder
- Salt to taste

For Guacamole:
- 2 ripe avocados, mashed
- 1 tomato, diced
- ¼ cup red onion, finely chopped
- 1 lime, juiced

- Salt and pepper to taste

For Assembly:
- Cooked rice
- Tortilla chips
- Fresh cilantro for garnish
- Lime wedges

Instructions:

Sauté Fajita Vegetables:
- Sliced bell peppers and red onion should be softened by cooking them in olive oil in a pan. After tossing the veggies with fajita spice, fry them until they are crisp-tender.

Prepare the Black Beans:
- Heat the Black Beans with the Cumin, Chili Powder, and Salt in a small saucepan. Cook until well heated.

- To prepare guacamole, mash avocados, diced tomato, chopped red onion, lime juice, salt, and pepper in a basin. Blend well to make guacamole.

Assemble Fajita Bowl:
 - Combine cooked rice, seasoned black beans, fajita veggies, and a dollop of guacamole in bowls. Add lime wedges, fresh cilantro, and tortilla chips as garnish.

8. Pumpkin and Sage Risotto

Ingredients:

- 1 cup Arborio rice
- ½ cup dry white wine
- 4 cups vegetable broth, warmed
- 1 cup canned pumpkin puree
- ½ cup Parmesan cheese, grated
- ¼ cup fresh sage leaves, chopped
- 1 onion, finely chopped
- 2 tablespoons butter
- 2 tablespoons olive oil
- Salt and black pepper to taste

Instructions:

- To sauté onion and sage, place chopped onion and fresh sage in a big skillet with butter and olive oil. Cook until the onion becomes transparent.

Toast Arborio Rice:
- Place the Arborio rice in the pan and let it cook for one to two minutes, or until it begins to become golden brown.

Use Wine to Deglaze the Pan:
- Add the white wine and stir until the wine is mostly absorbed.

Add Pumpkin and Broth:
- Add one ladle at a time, stir in the pumpkin puree and then slowly pour in the heated vegetable broth. Before adding more, let the previous additions soak. Keep going until the rice is cooked through and creamy.

Finish with Cheese:

- Add grated Parmesan cheese, stir, and allow it to melt into the risotto after seasoning with salt and black pepper.

Serve:

- Serve the Pumpkin and Sage Risotto hot, garnished with additional sage leaves and a sprinkle of Parmesan.

9. Vegetarian Spinach and Artichoke Stuffed Shells

Ingredients:

- 20 jumbo pasta shells, cooked according to package instructions
- 2 cups ricotta cheese
- 1 cup frozen chopped spinach, thawed and drained
- 1 can (14 oz) artichoke hearts, drained and chopped
- 1 cup mozzarella cheese, shredded
- ½ cup Parmesan cheese, grated

- 2 cloves garlic, minced
- 1 egg
- 2 cups marinara sauce
- Salt and black pepper to taste
- Fresh basil for garnish

Instructions:

Prepare filling:
   - Combine ricotta cheese, chopped artichoke hearts, chopped spinach, mozzarella, Parmesan, minced garlic, and beaten egg in a bowl. Put some salt and black pepper over it.

Stuff Shells:
 - Spoon the spinach and artichoke mixture into each cooked pasta shell.

 Bake:
- Transfer the filled shells into an ovenproof plate. Dollop with marinara sauce. Bake for approximately 25 to 30 minutes, or until the

shells are well cooked, at 375°F (190°C) in the oven.

Garnish and Serve:
- Sprinkle the vegetarian spinach and artichoke stuffed shells with freshly chopped basil and serve them hot.

Chapter 11

Snacks, Desserts, and Side Dishes

Healthy Snack Recipes:

1. Greek Yogurt Parfait

Ingredients:

- 1 cup Greek yogurt
- ½ cup granola
- ½ cup mixed berries (strawberries, blueberries, raspberries)
- 1 tablespoon honey
- 1 tablespoon chia seeds (optional)
- ¼ cup chopped nuts (almonds, walnuts)

Instructions:

Layer Granola and Yogurt:
 - Arrange the granola and Greek yogurt in a glass or dish.

Add Berries:
 - Cover the yogurt and granola with a layer of mixed berries.

Drizzle Honey:
 - To add sweetness, drizzle honey over the berries.

Sprinkle Nuts and Chia Seeds:
 - You may optionally top with chopped nuts and sprinkle chia seeds for extra nourishment.

Repeat Layers:
 - Continue layering until the top of the bowl or glass is reached.

2. Apple Slices with Almond Butter

Ingredients:

- 2 apples, cored and sliced
- ¼ cup almond butter
- 2 tablespoons honey
- ½ teaspoon cinnamon
- ¼ cup granola (optional)
- Sliced almonds for garnish

Instructions:

- To make apple slices, core and thinly slice the apples.

Apply Almond Butter:
- Apply a thin layer of almond butter to every apple slice.

Drizzle Honey and Sprinkle Cinnamon:
- To enhance the flavor of the almond butter, drizzle honey over it.

Optional Granola Topping:

  - You may top the almond butter with granola for an extra crunch.

Garnish:

  - To provide an additional layer of texture, scatter sliced almonds on top.

Serve:

  - Put the apple slices and almond butter on a platter and start serving right away.

3. Vegetable Sticks with Hummus

Ingredients:

- Carrot sticks
- Celery sticks
- Cucumber sticks
- Cherry tomatoes
- 1 cup hummus

Instructions:

- To prepare the vegetables, wash and chop the cherry tomatoes, cucumber, celery, and carrot sticks.

Serve with Hummus:
- Put the veggie sticks on a platter and provide a cup of hummus so that guests may dip into it.

4. Trail Mix with Nuts and Dried Fruits

Ingredients:

- 1 cup almonds
- 1 cup walnuts
- 1 cup cashews
- ½ cup pumpkin seeds
- ½ cup dried cranberries
- ½ cup raisins
- ½ cup dark chocolate chips
- ½ teaspoon sea salt

Instructions:

For the Roast Nuts and Seeds:
- Set the oven's temperature to 350°F (180°C). Almonds, walnuts, cashews, and pumpkin seeds should all be gently toasted after 8 to 10 minutes of roasting on a baking pan.

Combine with Dried Fruits:
- Place the roasted nuts and seeds, raisins, and dark chocolate chips in a big bowl.

Add Salt Seasoning:
- Dredge the trail mix in sea salt and stir thoroughly.

Chill and Store:
- Before putting the trail mix in an airtight container to be stored, let it chill fully.

Serve:

 - As a healthy snack for energy on-the-go, serve the Trail Mix with Nuts and Dried Fruits.

5. Roasted Chickpeas

Ingredients:

- 2 cans (15 oz each) chickpeas, drained and rinsed
- 2 tablespoons olive oil
- 1 teaspoon smoked paprika
- 1 teaspoon cumin
- ½ teaspoon garlic powder
- ½ teaspoon onion powder
- ½ teaspoon cayenne pepper (optional)
- Salt to taste

Instructions:

Oven Prep:

- Set the oven's temperature to 400°F, or 200°C.

- Pat dry the chickpeas using a paper towel to get rid of any extra moisture.

- Toss the chickpeas with olive oil, cumin, smoked paprika, onion powder, garlic powder, cayenne pepper (if using), and salt in a bowl.

- Arrange the seasoned chickpeas in a single layer on a baking sheet. Roast for 25 to 30 minutes, or until crispy and golden.

6. Cottage Cheese with Pineapple

Ingredients:

- 1 cup cottage cheese
- 1 cup fresh pineapple, diced
- 2 tablespoons honey
- ¼ cup chopped mint (optional)

Instructions:

Mix Pineapple and Cottage Cheese:
- Place fresh pineapple and cottage cheese in a bowl.

Drizzle with Honey:
 - Drizzle the pineapple and cottage cheese mixture with honey.

Add Mint (Selective):
  - You may add chopped mint to the top for an extra cool taste.

Serve:
 - For a filling and light snack or breakfast alternative, serve chilled cottage cheese and pineapple.

7. Edamame with Sea Salt

Ingredients:

- 2 cups frozen edamame
- ½ tablespoon sea salt

Instructions:

Boil Edamame:
  - Bring a pot of water to a boil and cook frozen edamame for four to five minutes, or until they are soft.

Drain and Season:
  - While the edamame are still warm, drain them and throw them with sea salt.

8. Whole Grain Crackers with Avocado

Ingredients:

- Whole grain crackers
- 2 avocados, mashed
- 1 tablespoon lemon juice
- Salt and black pepper to taste
- Red pepper flakes for garnish (optional)

Instructions:

- To make avocado mash, mash the avocados with lemon juice, salt, and black pepper in a bowl.

Spread on Crackers:
- Top whole grain crackers with the avocado mixture.

Optional Garnish:
- For an optional spicy touch, top with red pepper flakes.

Serve:

- As an easy and wholesome snack, serve Whole Grain Crackers with Avocado.

9. Kale Chips

Ingredients:

- 1 bunch kale, stems removed and leaves torn into bite-sized pieces
- 1 tablespoon olive oil
- ½ teaspoon sea salt
- ½ teaspoon garlic powder
- ¼ teaspoon black pepper

Instructions:

Oven Prep:
- Set the oven's temperature to 350°F, or 180°C.

Massage the kale leaves:

- In a bowl, massage the kale leaves until fully coated with olive oil, sea salt, garlic powder, and black pepper.

Bake:
- Arrange the kale pieces on a baking sheet in a single layer. Bake until the edges are crispy, 10 to 15 minutes.

Chill and Savor:
- Let the Kale Chips chill down before savoring them as a tasty and crispy snack.

10. Smoothie Bowl

Ingredients:

- 1 cup frozen mixed berries (strawberries, blueberries, raspberries)
- 1 ripe banana, sliced and frozen
- ½ cup Greek yogurt

- ½ cup spinach leaves
- ½ cup almond milk
- 1 tablespoon chia seeds
- Toppings: sliced fresh fruits, granola, shredded coconut, and a drizzle of honey

Instructions:

Prepare Frozen Fruits:
 - To get a thick and creamy consistency, make sure the banana slices and berries are frozen ahead.

Blend Smoothie Base:
 - Place frozen banana slices, Greek yogurt, chia seeds, frozen berries, and almond milk in a blender.

Blend till Smooth:
 - Process the mixture in a blender until it's creamy and smooth. If additional almond milk is required to get the right consistency, add it.

Transfer to a Bowl:
- Transfer the smoothie to a bowl.

Add Toppings:
- Sprinkle granola, shredded coconut, honey, and fresh fruit slices on top of the smoothie bowl.

Nutrient-Rich Desserts:

1. Fresh Fruit Salad

Ingredients:

- 2 cups watermelon, diced
- 1 cup pineapple, diced
- 1 cup strawberries, hulled and halved
- 1 cup grapes, halved
- 1 banana, sliced
- 1 kiwi, peeled and sliced
- 1 tablespoon fresh mint leaves, chopped (optional)
- Juice of 1 lime

Instructions:

-   Fruit preparation includes chopping pineapple and watermelon, peeling and slicing kiwis, hulling and halving strawberries, and halving grapes.

Combine Fruits:
- Place all of the prepped fruits in a big bowl.

Add the optional fresh mint:
- You may optionally top the fruit salad with chopped fresh mint.

Drizzle with Lime Juice:
- To add a zesty, refreshing taste to the fruit salad, drizzle with lime juice.

Gently Toss:
- Toss the fruit salad gently until it's well incorporated.

2. Dark Chocolate-Dipped Strawberries

Ingredients:

- 1 cup dark chocolate chips
- 1 tablespoon coconut oil
- 12 large strawberries, washed and dried

Instructions:

- To prepare the strawberries, make sure they are thoroughly dry and clean.

Melt Chocolate:
- In a bowl that is safe to use in the microwave, melt dark chocolate chips with coconut oil, stirring every 20 seconds, until smooth.

Dip Strawberries:
- Holding each strawberry by the stem, dip it about two thirds of the way into the melted chocolate.

Place on Parchment:
 - Arrange the dipped strawberries on a dish covered with parchment paper.

Chill:
 - Place the strawberries dipped in dark chocolate in the refrigerator to cool for 15 to 20 minutes, or until the chocolate solidifies.

3. Yogurt Parfait with Nuts and Seeds

Ingredients:

- 1 cup Greek yogurt
- ½ cup granola
- ¼ cup mixed nuts (almonds, walnuts), chopped
- 2 tablespoons chia seeds
- 1 tablespoon honey
- Fresh berries for garnish

Instructions:

Layer Granola and Yogurt:
- Arrange the granola and Greek yogurt in a glass or dish.

Add Nuts and Seeds:
- Top the yogurt and granola with chopped chia seeds and mixed nuts.

Drizzle Honey:
- To add sweetness, drizzle honey over top.

Garnish with Berries:
- To add a pop of color and taste, garnish the yogurt parfait with fresh berries.

Serve:
- For a filling and healthy breakfast or snack, serve this healthy yogurt parfait with nuts and seeds.

4. Baked Apples with Cinnamon

Ingredients:

- 4 medium-sized apples, cored
- ¼ cup raisins
- ¼ cup chopped nuts (walnuts or pecans)
- 2 tablespoons maple syrup
- 1 teaspoon ground cinnamon
- ¼ teaspoon nutmeg
- 1 tablespoon melted butter or coconut oil

Instructions:

Oven Prep:
 - Set the oven's temperature to 375°F, or 190°C.

Prepare the apples:
 - Core the fruit, being sure to save the bottoms. Put them inside a dish for baking.

Mix Filling:
- Combine chopped nuts, melted butter or coconut oil, ground cinnamon, nutmeg, raisins, and maple syrup in a bowl.

Fill Apples:
- Insert the raisin and nut mixture into each cored apple.

Bake:
- Bake the stuffed apples for around 25 to 30 minutes, or until they are soft, in a preheated oven.

- To serve, top the warm baked apples with cinnamon with a dollop of Greek yogurt or a scoop of vanilla ice cream.

5. Chia Pudding with Berries

Ingredients:

- ¼ cup chia seeds
- 1 cup almond milk (or any milk of choice)

- 1 tablespoon honey or maple syrup
- ½ teaspoon vanilla extract
- Mixed berries for topping

Instructions:

Combine Chia Pudding Base:
 - In a bowl, blend together almond milk, vanilla extract, honey or maple syrup, and chia seeds. Mix well to blend.

Refrigerate:
 - To help the chia pudding solidify, cover the bowl and place it in the fridge for at least four hours or overnight.

Toss and Serve:
 - Give the chia pudding a thorough toss just before serving. To get the right consistency, add extra milk as needed.

Add Berries on Top:
 - Transfer the chia pudding into serving dishes and garnish with a mixture of berries.

Serve:

- For a tasty and nourishing dessert or brunch, serve cold Chia Pudding with Berries.

6. Avocado Chocolate Mousse

Ingredients:

- 2 ripe avocados, peeled and pitted
- ¼ cup cocoa powder
- ¼ cup maple syrup or honey
- ¼ cup almond milk (or any milk of choice)
- 1 teaspoon vanilla extract
- Pinch of salt

Instructions:

Ingredients to be blended:
- Place avocados, cocoa powder, almond milk, vanilla extract, maple syrup or honey,

and a dash of salt in a blender or food processor and mix until smooth.

- To help the avocado chocolate mousse firm up, place it in the refrigerator for at least two hours.

- Arrange the chilled Avocado Chocolate Mousse into glasses or bowls for serving. Add some chocolate powder or fresh berries as a garnish, if desired.

7. Nut and Seed Energy Balls: Frozen Banana Bites

Ingredients:

- 2 bananas, peeled and sliced
- ¼ cup peanut butter or almond butter
- ¼ cup dark chocolate chips
- 1 tablespoon coconut oil
- Toppings: shredded coconut, chopped nuts, or chia seeds (optional)

Instructions:

- To prepare the banana slices, slice them into rounds and arrange them on a dish coated with parchment paper.

Assemble Banana Sandwiches:
- On half of the banana slices, spread a little quantity of almond or peanut butter. Place the remaining banana slices on top to make "sandwiches."

Melt Chocolate:
- Using coconut oil and dark chocolate chips in a dish that is safe to microwave, stir until smooth, melting the chocolate every 20 seconds.

Dip Banana Bites:
- Evenly cover each banana "sandwich" by dipping it into the melted chocolate.

Optionally Add Toppings:
- You may choose to top the chocolate-coated banana nibbles with chopped almonds, chia seeds, or shredded coconut.

Freeze:
- Allow the banana bits to solidify in the freezer for a minimum of two hours.

8. Quinoa Pudding with Coconut Milk

Ingredients:

- 1 cup cooked quinoa
- 1 cup coconut milk
- 2 tablespoons honey or maple syrup
- ½ teaspoon vanilla extract
- ¼ teaspoon cinnamon
- Fresh berries for topping

Instructions:

Mixing the Ingredients: - Place the cooked quinoa, coconut milk, cinnamon, vanilla essence, honey, or maple syrup in a saucepan.

Simmer:
- Slowly cook the mixture over low heat, stirring now and again, until it thickens and becomes pudding-like.

Chill:
- To enjoy the Quinoa Pudding cold, let it come to room temperature or store it in the refrigerator.

Add Berries on Top:
- Transfer the quinoa pudding into serving dishes and garnish with raw berries.

Serve:
- Offer Quinoa Pudding with Coconut Milk as a filling, high-protein breakfast or dessert.

9. Papaya Boat with Lime

Ingredients:

- 1 ripe papaya, halved and seeds removed
- Juice of 1 lime
- Fresh mint leaves for garnish (optional)

Instructions:

- To prepare the papaya halves, cut a ripe one in half and scoop out the seeds.

Squeeze Lime Juice:
- Drizzle each half of a papaya with lime juice.

Optional Garnish:
  - For an extra touch of freshness, feel free to garnish with fresh mint leaves.

10. Nut and Seed Energy Balls

Ingredients:

- 1 cup nuts (almonds, cashews, or a mix), toasted
- ½ cup dates, pitted
- 2 tablespoons chia seeds
- 2 tablespoons flax seeds
- 2 tablespoons nut butter (peanut butter, almond butter)
- ½ teaspoon vanilla extract
- Pinch of salt
- Desiccated coconut for coating (optional)

Instructions:

- Process dates, roasted almonds, chia seeds, flaxseeds, nut butter, vanilla essence, and a little amount of salt in a food processor until a sticky dough forms.

- Take tiny spoonfuls of the mixture and roll them into balls of energy.

Apply a Coconut Coat (Optional):
- For an additional layer of texture, feel free to roll the energy balls in desiccated coconut.

- To make the Nut and Seed Energy Balls firmer, chill them in the fridge for at least half an hour.

Sides dish Recipes

1. Roasted Vegetables

Ingredients:

- 3 cups mixed vegetables (carrots, bell peppers, zucchini, cherry tomatoes, etc.), chopped
- 2 tablespoons olive oil
- 1 teaspoon dried herbs (rosemary, thyme, or your choice)
- Salt and black pepper to taste

Instructions:

Oven Prep:
  - Set the oven's temperature to 400°F, or 200°C.

Vegetable Preparation:
  - Dice the mixed veggies into small pieces.

Drizzle with Oil and Herbs:

- In a dish, toss the veggies to cover them equally with a mixture of olive oil, dried herbs, salt, and black pepper.

Roast:

- Arrange the oiled veggies in a single layer on a baking sheet. Roast for 20 to 25 minutes, or until they are soft and brown, in a preheated oven.

2. Quinoa Pilaf

Ingredients:

- 1 cup quinoa, rinsed
- 2 cups vegetable broth or water
- 1 tablespoon olive oil
- 1 onion, finely chopped
- 2 cloves garlic, minced
- 1 cup mixed vegetables (peas, carrots, corn)
- Salt and black pepper to taste
- Fresh parsley for garnish (optional)

Instructions:

- To cook quinoa, put it in a pot with water or vegetable broth. After bringing to a boil, lower the heat, cover the pot, and simmer the quinoa for fifteen minutes, or until the liquid has been absorbed.

Sauté Vegetables:
- Heat olive oil in a different pan. Chopped onion and garlic should be sautéed until tender. When the mixed veggies are crisp-tender, add them and simmer.

Mix Quinoa and veggies:
- Combine sautéed veggies with cooked quinoa. Put some salt and black pepper over it.

Garnish and Serve:
- If preferred, sprinkle fresh parsley over the Quinoa Pilaf. Serve as a wholesome and adaptable side dish.

3. Kale and Walnut Salad

Ingredients:

- 4 cups kale, stemmed and chopped
- ½ cup walnuts, toasted and chopped
- ¼ cup dried cranberries
- ¼ cup feta cheese, crumbled
- 2 tablespoons olive oil
- 1 tablespoon balsamic vinegar
- 1 teaspoon honey
- Salt and black pepper to taste

Instructions:

- To prepare the kale, massage it with olive oil for several minutes to make it softer.

Assemble Salad:
- Combine crumbled feta cheese, roasted walnuts, dried cranberries, and massaged kale in a bowl.

Prepare Dressing:

- To prepare the dressing, whisk together olive oil, honey, balsamic vinegar, salt, and black pepper.

Drizzle Dressing:

- Pour the dressing into the kale salad and mix to ensure that it is uniformly coated.

4. Mashed Sweet Potatoes

Ingredients:

- 3 large sweet potatoes, peeled and cubed
- 2 tablespoons butter
- ¼ cup milk (dairy or plant-based)
- 1 tablespoon maple syrup
- ½ teaspoon ground cinnamon
- Salt to taste

Instructions:

Boil Sweet Potatoes:
 - Bring peeled and diced sweet potatoes to a fork-tender consistency by boiling them.

Mash Potatoes:
 - After draining, mash the sweet potatoes using a fork or potato masher.

Add Ingredients:
 - To the mashed sweet potatoes, add butter, milk, maple syrup, ground cinnamon, and salt. Blend and crush until homogenous.

Modify Consistency:
 - If necessary, add extra milk to modify the consistency.

5. Brussels Sprouts with Balsamic Glaze

Ingredients:

- 1 pound Brussels sprouts, trimmed and halved
- 2 tablespoons olive oil
- Salt and black pepper to taste
- 2 tablespoons balsamic glaze
- ¼ cup shaved Parmesan cheese (optional)

Instructions:

Oven Prep:
  - Set the oven's temperature to 400°F, or 200°C.

  - Prepare the Brussels sprouts by cutting them in half and trimming the ends.

Drizzle with Olive Oil:
 - Place Brussels sprouts in a basin and toss to coat equally with olive oil, salt, and black pepper.

Roast:
 - Arrange the Brussels sprouts in a single layer on a baking sheet. Roast for 20 to 25 minutes, or until brown and crispy, in an oven that has been prepared.

Drizzle Balsamic Glaze:
 - Drizzle the roasted Brussels sprouts with the balsamic glaze. Toss in the coat.

Parmesan Topping Option:
 - Before serving, if preferred, sprinkle some shaved Parmesan cheese on top.

6. Cauliflower Rice

Ingredients:

- 1 medium cauliflower, grated or processed into rice-like texture
- 2 tablespoons olive oil
- 2 cloves garlic, minced
- Salt and black pepper to taste
- Fresh parsley for garnish (optional)

Instructions:

- To make cauliflower rice, grate or pulse the cauliflower until it resembles little rice particles.

Sauté Garlic:
- Heat olive oil in a pan. Garlic, minced, and sauté until aromatic.

Prepare the Cauliflower Rice:
- Place the rice in the pan. Simmer for 5 to 7 minutes, stirring often, or until soft but not mushy.

- Use black pepper and salt to season the cauliflower rice.

- If preferred, garnish with fresh parsley.

- Cauliflower rice is a wholesome and low-carb substitute for regular rice.

7. Spinach and Mushroom Saute

Ingredients:

- 1 tablespoon olive oil
- 1 onion, finely chopped
- 2 cups mushrooms, sliced
- 4 cups fresh spinach leaves
- 2 cloves garlic, minced
- Salt and black pepper to taste
- Lemon juice for a fresh finish

Instructions:

Sauté the onion and mushrooms:
 - Heat the olive oil in a pan. Add the sliced mushrooms and simmer until they shed their moisture after sautéing the minced onion until it becomes transparent.

Add Garlic and Spinach:
   - Add minced garlic and fresh spinach leaves to the pan. Sauté the spinach until it wilts.

Season:
 - Add salt and black pepper to the spinach and mushroom combination.

Add a Squeeze of Lemon Juice:
   - To give the sauté a crisp, colorful finish, squeeze some lemon juice over it.

8. Quinoa and Black Bean Stuffed Peppers

Ingredients:

- 4 large bell peppers, halved and seeds removed
- 1 cup quinoa, cooked
- 1 can (15 oz) black beans, drained and rinsed
- 1 cup corn kernels (fresh or frozen)
- 1 cup diced tomatoes
- 1 teaspoon ground cumin
- 1 teaspoon chili powder
- Salt and black pepper to taste
- 1 cup shredded cheese (cheddar or Mexican blend)
- Fresh cilantro for garnish (optional)

Instructions:

Oven Prep:
- Set the oven's temperature to 375°F, or 190°C.

Prepare the Peppers:
  - Cut the bell peppers in half and take out the seeds. Put them inside a dish for baking.

Mix Filling:
  - Place cooked quinoa, black beans, corn, diced tomatoes, chili powder, ground cumin, salt, and black pepper in a dish.

Stuffed Peppers:
  - Stuff the black bean and quinoa mixture into each pepper half.

Add Cheese on Top:
  - Drizzle the filled peppers with shredded cheese.

Bake:
  - Bake the peppers for 25 to 30 minutes, or until they are soft, in a preheated oven.

Garnish (Optional):
  - If preferred, garnish with fresh cilantro.

9. Asparagus with Lemon Zest

Ingredients:

- 1 bunch asparagus, trimmed
- 2 tablespoons olive oil
- Zest of 1 lemon
- Salt and black pepper to taste
- Lemon wedges for serving

Instructions:

Oven Prep:
 - Set the oven's temperature to 400°F, or 200°C.

Toss the Asparagus:
  - Place the trimmed asparagus in a baking dish and toss with olive oil, lemon zest, salt, and black pepper.

Roast:
 - Roast the asparagus for 10 to 12 minutes, or until it's crisp-tender. Preheat the oven.

10.Baked Eggplant Slices

Ingredients

- 1 large eggplant, sliced into rounds
- 2 tablespoons olive oil
- 1 teaspoon dried Italian herbs (basil, oregano, thyme)
- Salt and black pepper to taste
- 1 cup marinara sauce
- 1 cup shredded mozzarella cheese
- Fresh basil for garnish (optional)

Instructions:

Oven Prep:
- Set the oven's temperature to 375°F, or 190°C.

- Prepare the eggplant by slicing it into rounds and arranging it on a baking pan.

Oil Brushing:
 - Lightly coat the eggplant slices on both sides with extra virgin olive oil. Season with salt, black pepper, and dried Italian herbs.

Bake:
 - Bake the eggplant for 15 to 20 minutes, or until it's soft, in a preheated oven.

Add Marinara and Cheese on Top:
 - Drizzle each eggplant slice with marinara sauce and sprinkle shredded mozzarella cheese on top.

Broil:
 - Continue broiling the cheese for a further three to five minutes, or until it is melted and bubbling.

Garnish (Optional):
 - If preferred, garnish with fresh basil.

11. Garlic Parmesan Roasted Broccoli

Ingredients:

- 1 pound broccoli florets
- 3 tablespoons olive oil
- 4 cloves garlic, minced
- ¼ cup grated Parmesan cheese
- 1 teaspoon lemon zest
- Salt and black pepper to taste

Instructions:

Oven Prep:
  - Set the oven's temperature to 425°F (220°C).

Toss Broccoli:
  - Combine olive oil, minced garlic, Parmesan cheese, lemon zest, salt, and black pepper in a bowl with the broccoli florets.

Roast:

- Arrange the broccoli that has been coated in a single layer on a baking sheet. Bake for 20 to 25 minutes, or until the edges become crispy, in a preheated oven.

12. Cilantro Lime Rice

Ingredients:

- 1 cup long-grain white rice
- 2 cups water or vegetable broth
- ¼ cup fresh cilantro, chopped
- Juice of 1 lime
- Salt to taste

Instructions:

Cook Rice:
- Use water or vegetable broth to cook white rice in a rice cooker or on the stovetop.

Fluff Rice:
- Use a fork to fluff the cooked rice.

Add the Lime and Cilantro:
- Add the lime juice and chopped cilantro.
To taste, add salt.

13. Sautéed Garlic Mushrooms

Ingredients:

- 1 pound mushrooms, sliced
- 2 tablespoons butter
- 3 cloves garlic, minced
- 2 tablespoons fresh parsley, chopped
- Salt and black pepper to taste

Instructions:

- To sauté mushrooms, melt butter in a pan over medium heat. Sliced mushrooms should be added and sautéed until they release moisture.

- Saute the minced garlic in the mushrooms until it becomes aromatic.

- Use black pepper and salt to season the garlic mushrooms.

- Add freshly cut parsley to finish.

14. Caprese Salad

Ingredients:

- 4 large tomatoes, sliced
- 1 pound fresh mozzarella cheese, sliced
- Fresh basil leaves
- 3 tablespoons extra-virgin olive oil
- Balsamic glaze for drizzling
- Salt and black pepper to taste

Instructions:

- To assemble the salad, place tomato and mozzarella slices in succession on a serving dish.

Add the Basil Leaves:
 - Place a few fresh basil leaves in between the slices of mozzarella and tomato.

Drizzle with Olive Oil:
 - Drizzle the salad with extra-virgin olive oil. Put some salt and black pepper over it.

Add Balsamic Glaze as a Finish:
 - Drizzle the caprese salad with a balsamic glaze.

15. Lemon Herb Roasted Potatoes

Ingredients:

- 2 pounds baby potatoes, halved
- 3 tablespoons olive oil
- 2 tablespoons fresh herbs (rosemary, thyme, or a mix), chopped
- Zest of 1 lemon
- Salt and black pepper to taste

Instructions:

Oven Prep:
 - Set the oven's temperature to 425°F (220°C).

Coat Potatoes:
 - Combine olive oil, chopped herbs, lemon zest, salt, and black pepper in a dish and toss to coat the halved young potatoes.

Roast:
 - Arrange the potatoes that have been coated on a baking sheet. Roast for 30 to 35 minutes, or until crispy and brown, in a preheated oven.

16. Buttered Corn with Chili and Lime

Ingredients:

- 4 cups corn kernels (fresh or frozen)
- 2 tablespoons unsalted butter
- 1 teaspoon chili powder

- Juice of 1 lime
- Salt to taste
- Fresh cilantro for garnish (optional)

Instructions:

Cook Corn:
  - Thaw frozen corn if using it. Boil or steam fresh corn until it becomes soft.

Butter and Spice:
  - Melt butter in a skillet over medium heat. Stir in corn, salt, and chili powder. Fry for three to five minutes.

Add a last touch of lime:
  - Drizzle the corn with lime juice and toss to coat.

Garnish (Optional):
  - If preferred, garnish with fresh cilantro.

17. Mashed Cauliflower with Garlic and Chives

Ingredients:

- 1 large head cauliflower, cut into florets
- 2 tablespoons butter
- 3 cloves garlic, minced
- ¼ cup chopped fresh chives
- Salt and black pepper to taste

Instructions:

-    Steaming cauliflower florets will make them extremely soft.

Mash Cauliflower:
 - For a smoother texture, mash the cooked cauliflower with a potato masher or mix it.

Incorporate Flavor:
 - Melt butter in a pan. When aromatic, add the minced garlic and sauté it. Stir into the cauliflower mash.

- Add the chopped chives and season. Put some salt and black pepper over it.

- As a low-carb substitute for mashed potatoes, serve mashed cauliflower with garlic and chives.

8. Balsamic Glazed Brussels Sprouts

Ingredients:

- 1 pound Brussels sprouts, trimmed and halved
- 2 tablespoons olive oil
- Salt and black pepper to taste
- 2 tablespoons balsamic glaze
- 1/4 cup shaved Parmesan cheese (optional)

Instructions:

Oven Prep:
- Set the oven's temperature to 400°F, or 200°C.

Toss Brussels Sprouts:
- Combine olive oil, salt, and black pepper and toss the sprouts. Transfer to a baking sheet.

Roast:
- Roast for 20 to 25 minutes, or until the edges are crispy, in an oven that has been prepared.

Drizzle with Balsamic Glaze:
- Drizzle the roasted Brussels sprouts with balsamic glaze. Toss in the coat.

Optional Parmesan Topping:
- Before serving, sprinkle some shaved Parmesan cheese on top.

19. Tomato and Avocado Salad

Ingredients:

- 4 large tomatoes, diced
- 2 ripe avocados, diced
- ¼ cup red onion, finely chopped
- 2 tablespoons fresh cilantro, chopped
- 2 tablespoons extra-virgin olive oil
- Juice of 1 lime
- Salt and black pepper to taste

Instructions:

- Chop the avocados and tomatoes into small pieces. Chop the cilantro and red onion finely.

Assemble the salad:
- Combine the tomatoes, avocados, red onion, and cilantro in a bowl.

Dress the Salad:
- Pour lime juice and extra virgin olive oil over the greens. Put some salt and black pepper over it.

Gently Toss:
- Toss the avocado and tomato salad gently so that it coats evenly.

20. Quinoa and Cranberry Pilaf

Ingredients:

- 1 cup quinoa, rinsed
- 2 cups vegetable broth or water
- ½ cup dried cranberries
- ¼ cup chopped almonds
- 1 tablespoon olive oil
- 1 teaspoon orange zest
- Salt and black pepper to taste

Instructions:

- To cook quinoa, put it in a pot with water or vegetable broth. After bringing to a boil, lower the heat, cover, and simmer the quinoa for 15 minutes, or until it is tender.

Fluff Quinoa:
- Use a fork to fluff the cooked quinoa.

Add Almonds and Cranberries:
- Stir in chopped almonds, olive oil, orange zest, salt, and black pepper. Also add dried cranberries.

Toss and Serve:
- Gently toss the quinoa and cranberry pilaf, then serve it as a tasty, nutrient-dense side dish.

Conclusion:

Empowering Individuals for Long-Term Health

Knowing the significant role nutrition plays in breast cancer becomes a lighthouse on the way to heath, directing people toward making wise decisions. The goal of this book, "Breast Cancer Diet for the Newly Diagnosed," is to empower readers for long-term, maintained health in addition to offering insights into the complex link between diet and breast cancer.

Empowering People

The knowledge provided on these pages acts as a compass, pointing people in the direction of taking charge of their health. Knowledge is the foundation of empowerment, and knowing how food decisions may affect both prevention and rehabilitation makes it a powerful tool. Adopting a diet customized to meet personal needs allows one to take an active role in their health, building resilience and a sense of control.

Promoting Ongoing Nutritional Awareness: Maintaining long-term health requires ongoing effort rather than a one-time investment. Maintaining sustained well-being mostly consists of promoting continued dietary awareness. Being aware of how nutrition is changing as we manage the challenges of everyday living becomes essential. With this knowledge, people are able to modify and improve the foods they eat, making sure they are in line with the most recent findings about breast cancer and general health.

This book aims to create a more profound relationship between people and their nutrition by encouraging awareness when making eating decisions. With the adoption of an anti-cancer diet, comprehension of the subtle differences between functional and dysfunctional foods, and skill in negotiating the intricacies of side effects, readers are furnished with an extensive arsenal for their culinary expedition.

Appendix:

This appendix serves as a practical resource, offering a collection of nutritious recipes and sample meal plans tailored to different stages of breast cancer treatment..

Sample Meal Plans for Different Stages of Treatment:

1. **Early Treatment Phase:**
   - **Breakfast**: Greek Yogurt Parfait with Mixed Berries and Granola
   - **Lunch**: Quinoa and Vegetable Salad with Grilled Chicken
   - **Dinner**: Baked Salmon with Dill Sauce, Roasted Sweet Potatoes, and Sautéed Spinach

2. **Mid-Treatment Phase:**
   - **Breakfast**: Spinach and Mushroom Omelette with Whole Grain Toast
   - **Lunch**: Lentil Soup with a Side of Quinoa Salad

- **Dinner**: Stir-Fried Tofu with Broccoli and Brown Rice

3. **Post-Treatment and Recovery Phase:**
   - **Breakfast**: Chia Pudding with Mixed Berries and Almond Milk
   - **Lunch**: Grilled Vegetable Wrap with Hummus
   - **Dinner**: Mediterranean Chickpea Salad with Grilled Shrimp

Recipes:

1. Chia Pudding with Mixed Berries and Almond Milk:
   - Ingredients:
     - Chia seeds
     - Mixed berries
     - Almond milk
     - Maple syrup
   - Method:
     - Mix chia seeds with almond milk, add berries, and sweeten with maple syrup.

2. Mediterranean Chickpea Salad with Grilled Shrimp:
   - Ingredients:
     - Chickpeas
     - Cherry tomatoes
     - Cucumber
     - Feta cheese
     - Grilled shrimp
   - Method:
        - Combine chickpeas, tomatoes, cucumber, feta, and grilled shrimp. Toss with olive oil.

3. Grilled Vegetable Wrap with Hummus:
   - Ingredients:
     - Mixed grilled vegetables (zucchini, bell peppers, eggplant)
     - Whole grain wrap
     - Hummus
     - Fresh herbs (parsley, mint)
   - Method:

- Fill a whole grain wrap with grilled vegetables, spread hummus, and sprinkle fresh herbs.

4. Lentil Soup with a Side of Quinoa Salad:

- Ingredients:
  - Lentils
  - Carrots
  - Celery
  - Quinoa salad (quinoa, cherry tomatoes, cucumber)
- Method:
  - Cook lentils with carrots and celery. Serve with a refreshing quinoa salad.

5. Baked Salmon with Dill Sauce, Roasted Sweet Potatoes, and Sautéed Spinach:

- Ingredients:
  - Salmon filets
  - Sweet potatoes
  - Spinach
  - Dill sauce (Greek yogurt, dill, lemon)

- Method:
 - Bake salmon, roast sweet potatoes, and sauté spinach. Serve with dill sauce.

Review Request

Your thoughts are highly valued by me! Please allow me to briefly discuss your experiences with the "Breast Cancer Diet Cookbook For Beginners" guidance with you. Your input will raise the caliber of the material and benefit readers who are similar to you. Thank you for your time and thoughts.

Warm Regards
Andrea T. Rockwell

CBHW050800260726
9798883960139

www.ingramcontent.com/pod-product-compliance
Lightning Source LLC
Chambersburg PA
CBHW050800260726
48660CB00004B/1176